THE
ADJUSTED
AMERICAN

THE ADJUSTED AMERICAN

Normal Neuroses in the Individual and Society

Snell Putney, Ph.D.
and Gail J. Putney, Ph.D.

PERENNIAL LIBRARY
Harper & Row, Publishers
New York, Evanston, San Francisco, London

For our children, Cindy and Greg
May they remain free spirits

This book was originally published under the title NORMAL NEUROSIS.

First HARPER COLOPHON edition published 1966 by Harper & Row, Publishers, Incorporated, New York.

First PERENNIAL LIBRARY edition published 1972.

STANDARD BOOK NUMBER: 06-080270-7

5-75

CONTENTS

PREFACE

This is not a book about *them* (whose foibles we can view with detachment or even a certain relish); it is a book about *us*—the normal, the adjusted of our society. Its basic concern is with certain neuroses which are normal in America, and with the means of escaping them.

The reader is thus well qualified to evaluate the adequacy of our analyses; he has but to check them against his own experience. But he must allow for an initial tendency to reject certain conclusions because they are uncomfortable, or to refuse to let himself comprehend them. Since this book discusses the neuroses prevalent among its readers it cannot but incite a certain resistance—indeed, we sought to escape many of our conclusions during the years we planned and prepared the manuscript.

Therefore, although this book could probably be read from cover to cover in five or six hours, such a reading would present ideas far faster than they could be assimilated and evaluated. If we could choose our reader's approach, we would have him read it a chapter at a time, with intervening periods for reflection and debate.

Some of the phenomena we describe may be uniquely American, some could probably be found in all urban-industrial societies, and some are presumably universal among men. But we prefer to avoid for the present the problem of determining how many of the analyses could be extended to cultures other than the one of greatest interest to the reader and to ourselves. The repetition of such phrases as "the adjusted American" is intended only to underscore the limits of the generalization, not to suggest that the phenomena described are necessarily peculiar to Americans.

The characters which illustrate our analyses are stick figures, kept simple so that each can exemplify a specific pattern of behavior. Only in this manner could points be considered one at a time and built one upon another. Using real people as illustrations would have necessitated discussing everything at once, for the normal individual compounds one misunderstanding with another and is involved to some degree in most of the neuroses described in the book. Any resemblance to specific persons results from the prevalence of the neuroses, not from attempts at portraiture.

Our conclusions regarding love, obligation, sexual desire, and the hunger for approval will seem radical to many. But we hope that the most radical feature of the analyses lies in their conceptual parsimony and theoretical integration. Conceptual parsimony has been one of our fundamental objectives, and we have tried to drop or to simplify hoary and sacrosanct concepts of the psychological tradition whenever they did not make a useful contribution to the analysis. We have endeavored to keep all of the analyses tightly integrated with the underlying theory, and to keep this theory both evident and unobtrusive. The roots of our approach lie in symbolic interactionist social psychology, psychoanalytic theory, cultural anthropology, and existential philosophy.

The text is annotated only in the case of direct reference to other writers. Our deeper debt to the thought of others is too complex and diverse to permit facile acknowledgment. Perhaps the simplest way to pay homage is to list the names we most often invoked as we argued over the manuscript: Charles H. Cooley, Sigmund Freud, Erich Fromm, Sören Kierkegaard, Robert Lindner, George Herbert Mead, Margaret Mead, Friedrich Nietzsche, David Riesman, Jean Paul Sartre, W. I. Thomas, and Benjamin Lee Whorf.

We owe a more specific debt to George Alexander Young, Jr., whose psychiatric heresies were the stimulation and the starting point for the study. Finally, we would like to express our gratitude to Eleanor F. Snell and to Charles Elkind, who had the patience to read the manuscript in its early stages and made many valuable stylistic suggestions. We are, of course, solely responsible for the final product.

Slate Rock   S. P.
Sioux Narrows, Ontario   G. J. P.

Insanity in individuals is something rare—but in groups, parties, nations, and epochs, it is the rule.

FRIEDRICH NIETZSCHE

I

THE CONFORMIST
IN AMERICA

Men in masses are gripped by personal troubles, but they are not aware of their true meaning and source.

C. WRIGHT MILLS

After a careful appraisal of Americans, an observer writes: "In that immense crowd which throngs the avenues to power in the United States, I found very few men who displayed that manly candor and masculine independence of opinion which frequently distinguished the Americans in former times. . . . When I survey this countless multitude of beings, shaped to each other's likeness . . . the sight of such universal uniformity saddens and chills me, and I am tempted to regret that state of society which has ceased to be . . . every citizen, being assimilated to all the rest, is lost in the crowd." [1] *

Familiar words! But they were not written by David Riesman, not even in the twentieth century. They were written by Comte Alexis de Tocqueville after his visit to the United States in 1831. He found much that he admired, but he recoiled from the "tyranny of the majority" which seemed to be engulfing this

---

* Superior numbers refer to a section of notes beginning on page 231.

1

country a quarter of a century before the Civil War.

De Tocqueville's reflections underscore the point that the American conformist is not, as many seem to believe, a new breed. Most Americans, influenced by the televised glorification of Western frontier life, think of their forebears as free spirits characterized by a crusty independence. But, except for the restless minority who moved the edge of the frontier westward, most early Americans were so tied to the life of small rural communities that they hardly perceived their bonds. A man is not free to do that which he cannot imagine doing, and if in the past Americans had a limited awareness of pressures to conform, it was only because they could not grasp the possibility of behaving in ways fundamentally different from those of their fellows. For that matter, when nonconformance occurred it was likely to be considered heretical or sinful and dealt with summarily—those who wax nostalgic about the individualism of the American past might recall that dissenters were whipped out of the early colonies.

The startling change in conformity in America is thus not in the degree of conformity, but in the general *consciousness* of conformity. Despite their provincial reputation, Americans are becoming a cosmopolitan people and can no longer view their particular way of life with the insularity that characterized their ancestors. The isolation which produced and sustained the narrow horizons of an earlier era has all but disappeared. Mass communication, rapid transportation, and the requirements of commerce have created a mobile people intimately acquainted with regional differences. Moreover, the bulk of the population now lives in cities, where social classes mingle, ethnic groups interact, and differences in life style are a matter of daily experience.

Nor is the American's awareness of diversity limited to variations within his own society. In the last half century three vast citizen armies have been sent abroad and hundreds of thousands of American civilians have gone into Europe, Asia, Africa, and Latin America. Other troops—and the Peace Corps—follow in their wake today. Like ancient Romans, Americans now man far-flung outposts at points determined by the exigencies of world trade and politics. And, of course, there is the ubiquitous American tourist.

Exposure to different, often exotic, modes of existence has made Americans more aware of the patterns in their own culture. The English-speaking student who struggles with French verb conjugations becomes conscious of English verb forms which he has never before recognized—although he has used them continuously since childhood. By an analogous process, the American who becomes familiar with other ways of living acquires a heightened awareness of the pattern of his own life. The age of cultural innocence is passing; the American is beginning to recognize the patterns to which he conforms.

Moreover, for a decade and more, social critics from David Riesman to Vance Packard to the Sunday supplement writers have presented to an ever-widening audience a portrait of the American as an "other-directed," status-seeking conformist. The American finds this portrait consistent with his new consciousness of conformity, but he is uncomfortable with the image. He was reared in a tradition which taught that the ideal man chose his life without bending his knee to convention, and the fact that his ancestors did not necessarily measure up to this ideal is beside the point. His concern is with the fact that *he* does not. He is troubled by a feeling that he has exchanged mastery of himself for a place in the faceless ranks of a mass society.

Such a negative attitude toward conformity is not universal. There were, for example, the European enclaves in the Orient, small islands of conscious and proudly maintained conformity to patterns that originated thousands of miles away. Somerset Maugham portrays vividly the English colonial official at his post on some muddy Southeast Asian river, wearing formal dinner dress every evening, opening in daily sequence the issues of the *Times* of London that arrive in month-old batches—preserving to the last possible detail and by ingenious means a way of life that was his very being. Such a man hardly finds conformity a matter for shame; on the contrary, he is proud of conforming to the culture of a group with which he intensely identifies.

Thus the American's discomfort on perceiving that he, too, conforms cannot be dismissed as an inevitable reaction. We must account for why he feels uneasy. Lacking the Englishman's sense of tradition, the American pictures the conformist not as a correct gentleman but rather as a vacuous sheep. But perhaps the major source of his discontent is the scanty reward he receives through conforming. If the pattern of his life fulfilled him, he would be inclined to cherish it. But a growing number of Americans express a sense of emptiness and discontent that sits oddly with the affluent complacency ascribed to them.

Some of the discontented have tried to embrace the emptiness they encounter in their lives. This is not a new phenomenon. In the early decades of this century disaffected young French and German intellectuals elevated "nothingness" to a prime value. Having experienced the destruction of old ideals and

The denial of ~~any basis for~~ The existence of
any basis for Knowledge or Truth.
THE CONFORMIST IN AMERICA 5

purposes, they made destruction itself an ideal and a purpose. They expressed their nihilism in a series of literary ventures and art exhibits, a notable example being the exhibition in Cologne where the public was invited to attack the exhibits with axes thoughtfully provided for the purpose. These disillusioned young men called themselves "Dadaist," their mid-century American counterparts called themselves "Beat." Finding the pattern of life empty and obscene, they enshrined emptiness and obscenity. Their cultural heirs are the disaffected who reject the very symbols of the "American Way of Life" for which the conformist reaches greedily.

Although many other Americans are uneasy about conforming, most have too large a stake in the prevailing culture to turn their backs on it in angry protest. They may enjoy an occasional rebellious spree, may envy what they imagine to be the sex life of the bohemian fringe. But they shrink from the nonconformist label, fearing loss of respectability even more than they regret the loss of individuality.

Besides, they doubt that the nonconformist has made a good bargain. They wonder if the bohemian is free to bathe or only not to bathe, and they smile knowingly when hearing of beards shaved off because a Founder's Day celebration has made beards respectable. The price of nonconformity seems great and the freedom gained little more than conformity turned inside out.

Thus the American who has become uneasy about a conformist is typically unwilling to become a nonconformist. And yet his discontent remains. It seems to him that conformity has diminished his enjoyment of life and of himself, but he does not see anything he can do about it.

The Invisible Strait Jacket

The dilemma in which the dissatisfied conformist finds himself is a false dilemma, deriving from a narrow conception of conformity. The typical American thinks of conformity as involving taste, dress, manners, and opinion. But such superficial and conscious conformity is not the real source of his discontent. At the heart of the problem lies a deeper conformity of which he is hardly aware: conformity to the unquestioned assumptions of his culture.

In every society certain things are regarded as "self-evident truths." Different societies make different assumptions about man and the universe, but within each society the great majority of the people conform unwittingly to the prevailing set of beliefs. Louis Wirth observed that "the most important thing . . . we can know about a man is what he takes for granted, and the most elemental and important facts about a society are those that are seldom debated and generally regarded as settled." [2] Such implicit assumptions are the premises from which thought begins, the starting point for any course of action.

For example, in a society in which the power of evil spirits is "obvious" beyond debate, the average man employs devices to placate or confuse evil spirits. He may conform rigidly to local custom or he may innovate and experiment with various types of demon baffles, but it would be literally unthinkable to him to try doing without them altogether. His thought and action start from the premise that demons exist. And he finds proof of the influence of evil spirits on men's lives, for he interprets every stroke of misfortune, from a hailstorm that ruins his crop to the sudden death of a friend, as *prima facie* evidence of the power of malevolent spirits.

Similarly, in a society where war is taken for

granted, the average man applauds the development of increasingly destructive weapons systems. He may recognize that the use of these weapons would probably mean the destruction of himself, his society, and perhaps the human race. But his thought starts from the premise that military force is essential to survival and he cannot conceive of other alternatives. It is literally unthinkable to him that disarmament may be the only solution, so he can only laud every development in weaponry and hope that somehow the weapons will never be used.

So long as the individual takes for granted the assumptions that prevail in his society, he is limited to those thoughts and actions which are conceivable in terms of these assumptions. To perceive other alternatives he must first break free of the preconceptions which limit his imagination.

The prerequisite to such a breakthrough is to become fully conscious of those beliefs which are so familiar that they are seldom remarked. The best chance of recognizing and questioning such basic preconceptions occurs when some fortuitous exception to the "obvious" draws attention to a hitherto unchallenged belief. The person who is able to resist the temptation to ignore such evidence is rewarded with sudden insight and a new perspective.

This process of insight through surprise can be seen in a humble example. Our son grew up with a Siamese cat and when he was about three the only other cat in his limited world was also Siamese. Both had blue eyes, like all their breed. One day he saw a Persian cat padding toward him, and in the manner of three-year-olds he squatted down on the sidewalk to get a better look. The Persian also sat, wrapped her tail around her feet and regarded the boy. Suddenly he jumped up and ran into the house shouting, "I saw a cat with yellow eyes, Mommy! A cat with yellow eyes!"

In the moment when our small son and the Persian cat were face to face, two things had occurred to the boy: he became aware that all cats do not have blue eyes, and he also became aware that until that moment he had believed that they did. *He became conscious of the belief he had taken for granted only in the moment of perceiving that it was false.* Excited with his new insight and struggling with its implications, he bombarded his mother with questions about the eyes of cats—questions that would never have occurred to him before. Precisely the same process of challenging exception, breakthrough, and stimulation can occur with profound and consequential beliefs.

But unless or until some "yellow-eyed cat" challenges the beliefs men take for granted, these beliefs remain unremarked and unassailable. They constitute the most basic and restraining type of conformity, an invisible strait jacket on thought and thus ultimately on action.

The American who is chagrined about his conformity in matters of taste and consumption remains generally oblivious of his conformity to preconceptions regarding human needs and human nature. Yet the pattern of his life is predicated on these assumptions, and the ultimate cause of his discontent is his uncritical conformance to inaccurate assumptions concerning what he is and what he needs.

Normalcy and Adjustment

Somewhat inconsistently, the very Americans who chafe at conformity are likely to seek adjustment. One of the prevailing assumptions which Americans have learned to take for granted is that anxiety is a product of inadequate adjustment. This may be the case, but it is equally likely that anxiety reflects inadequacies in the pattern to which the individual attempts to adjust. *The adjusted individual is one who is able to fit readily into the normal patterns of his society*, but *it cannot be taken for granted that one who is adjusted is psychologically healthy*. He can be superbly adjusted to his culture, normal in every respect, and yet not lead a full and satisfying life.

The word "normal" is used by Americans in several senses. It means average or typical, as in the observation that the normal age at high school graduation is eighteen. It is also used to mean natural, as when one says that it is normal for boys to be interested in girls. This dual usage reflects the assumption that the customary patterns of one's culture are the natural ways of humanity.

However, the typical behaviors of a human society are not natural in the sense that the typical behaviors of an anthill are natural. For instance, the ant satisfies its hunger by unlearned behaviors which are built into the very structure of its nervous system. It does not need to learn how to find food, or what it can eat. It simply acts on the basis of its instincts and need satisfaction generally results. An ant's behavior is natural: that is, it is inherent in the nature of the ant.

In contrast, the behaviors that seem natural to men are usually only habitual. Man has a great capacity to learn, precisely because he is not limited to inflexible instinctive responses. Because man lacks such built-in response patterns, however, he has no inherent natural way of behaving.

Normal human behavior, then, is not natural, but rather habitual behavior that over a period of time has become typical in a particular society. The person who seeks to adjust more fully to the normal behavior of his society in the belief that he is moving toward fulfillment is only wriggling inside a strait jacket of conventional assumptions. He is only becoming more typical.

In no society are the normal behaviors perfectly adapted to the satisfaction of all human needs. The adjusted members of any given society will satisfy some needs effectively, others inadequately. The extent to which the adjusted individual is capable of satisfying his needs depends on the efficacy of the normal means of need satisfaction to which he has adjusted. And his well-being depends on the degree to which he is able to satisfy his needs.

When normal behaviors leave him deprived, the adjusted individual is relatively helpless. In the first place, he does not have a clear idea of what he is seeking; he has learned a set of customs, not an understanding of human needs. In the second place, he has learned to take for granted deprivation in certain areas of his life.

Just as the behaviors the adjusted individual employs are nearly universal in his society, so also are the consequences of these behaviors. In societies where the traditional means of securing food are inadequate, hunger may be accepted as an inevitable part of life. To be hungry is unpleasant, but the adjusted member of such a society cannot imagine a world without hunger—unless it be some mythical land or heaven where the hungry ones of this existence will find ultimate fulfillment. The adjusted man in such a society may struggle to secure sufficient food by traditional means, but he is unlikely to devise radically different means which might bring an end to hunger, or even to adopt radically new techniques if someone points them out to him. (The difficulty of introducing new agricultural techniques, for example, is attested by agronomists in most underdeveloped countries.) In short, those deprivations which are normal (that is, typical of most of the population) assume the stature of an inevitably recurring fact of life.

The adjusted American regards famine as an unusual crisis, a problem which can and must be resolved immediately. But in other areas of human need he is resigned to deprivation. For example, he accepts as a natural and inevitable part of life debilitating self-doubts and fears of personal inadequacy which are no more inevitable than starvation. He experiences this chronic deprivation simply because the normal behaviors and understandings of his society do not lead to fulfillment of his need for self-acceptance.

Neurosis may be defined as an internal, nonorganic barrier to need fulfillment. The adjusted American's difficulties in satisfying his emotional needs are not external, nor are they based in his organic nature; they are simply neuroses. These neuroses which plague the adjusted American and give a distinctive cast to American society are normal, just as "normal" malnutrition plagues and shapes other societies. It is the abnormal (i.e., nontypical) neuroses which invite attention and analysis because of their novelty; the normal neuroses are generally endured, precisely because of their prevalence in a society.

Autonomy

Given sufficient self-understanding to make a valid choice, most people would presumably choose to act in ways which lead to satisfaction. They would hardly be opposed to conformance *per se*, but they would seek to transcend adjustment to those beliefs and behaviors which leave their compatriots unsatisfied.

Those who are capable of conforming when conformance is functional, and also capable of real innovation (rather than mere nonconformance) when normal behaviors would leave them deprived, are *autonomous* in the fullest sense of the word. *Autonomy means the capacity of the individual to make valid choices of his behavior in the light of his needs.* To the extent that his choices are limited externally (by coercion) or internally (by normal neurosis or sterile rebellion) the individual is incapable of autonomy. In the case of most Americans, the internal limitations far outweigh the external ones.

In *The Lonely Crowd*, David Riesman uses the term *autonomy* in a similar sense. Pointing to autonomy as an ultimate goal, Riesman offers scant hope that it can be readily achieved. The institutional barriers, "false personalization" and "enforced privatization," appear to be too great, the way to autonomy too ill defined. But he does see some evidence of progress toward autonomy in the "other-directed" American who is concerned with being acceptable to the "jury of his peers" and thus is led to be increasingly self-conscious. According to Riesman, this awareness of self may ultimately lead to an "organic development of autonomy out of other-direction." [3]

If awareness of self is to lead toward autonomy, it must begin with awareness of the needs which motivate the self and of the normal neuroses which inhibit satisfaction of these needs. Such awareness may have the effect of an encounter with a "yellow-eyed cat" in suggesting alternative understandings and alternative means by which the individual can find satisfaction. Through such a process, self-awareness may enable the individual to transcend adjustment and move toward autonomy.

THE SQUIRREL CAGE

In therapy, our objective may be to restore the person's social adjustment and his "normal" neurotic tendencies. However, a more extensive objective would be a correction of all neurotic traits, even those condoned as "normal." LEWIS R. WOLBERG

The adjusted American does not recognize the neurotic nature of much of his behavior, because this behavior is normal. Taking conventional behaviors for granted, he merely redoubles his efforts when he fails to achieve relief from the tensions that drive him. Most of his fellows are running hard and he runs too, without asking where he is going—or why. (Each day the squirrel endeavors to run a little faster in his treadmill, confident that one day he will move ahead.)

The pattern of normal neurosis in which the adjusted American is trapped involves three basic elements: (1) faulty interpretation of human needs, (2) maladaptive behavior, which we shall term *misdirection*, and (3) chronic anxiety, the tension which accompanies deprivation.

Faulty Interpretation

The assumptions about human nature which are taken for granted by most Americans range from unsystematic but insightful folk wisdom to crippling misconceptions. In the following chapter we shall describe the needs which underlie human motivation; at this point our concern is in showing how faulty interpretation of needs can contribute to neurosis.

One of the most common forms of faulty interpretation of needs is particularization. *Particularization is the equation of some specific means of need satisfaction with the need itself.* The genesis of particularization is habit, or conditioned response. A person who has satisfied a need in one particular way since childhood is likely to have only a vague awareness of the need; his vivid consciousness will be of the familiar means of satisfaction. When feeling needful, he thinks instantly of the usual mode of fulfillment, bypassing recognition of the need itself. The effect is to confine his understanding to a specific pattern of response.

So long as the habitual means of meeting a need are adequate and readily available, there is no problem. When the person experiences need, he seeks that which fulfills it, an altogther functional and convenient pattern.

But if for any reason the habitual behaviors are not very effective—as in many cases they are not—particularization renders it difficult for the individual to recognize this fact, or to conceive of other techniques for meeting his need. Habit prevails, and he tends simply to try again in the familiar way. The result is analogous to bailing a boat with a sieve.

Even when the customary means of seeking satisfaction work well, there is the possibility that these may at some time become suddenly unavailable. The person with a particularized understanding of his need is then in serious trouble, for his ability to improvise and innovate is limited by his failure to perceive the broad, underlying need. To take an extreme example, men learn to satisfy their thirst by *drinking* liquids, a highly satisfying method. But many a shipwrecked sailor drifting without fresh water has died of thirst without recognizing the possibility of *chewing* the juices from raw fish.

Failing to comprehend that behind his usual satisfaction lies a basic need which could be fulfilled by unfamiliar means, the deprived person engages in exhausting but futile attempts to secure a form of satisfaction that is no longer available. Thus particularization is a potentially neurotic behavior, for it can become an internal barrier to need fulfillment.

The adjusted American has a particularized conception of many of his physical needs, from the foods he considers edible to the position in which he finds it easy to copulate. But it is particularization of his emotional needs (which we shall later deal with more specifically as *self* needs) which most frequently leads him into neurosis.

Faulty interpretation of needs may take other forms, such as the confusion of one need for another (e.g., a lonely person may interpret his craving as hunger and stuff himself insatiably because he is trying to satisfy the wrong need); or even confusion about *whose* need is felt. All of these faulty interpretations of need will be discussed in later chapters. In each case the individual has difficulty in finding satisfaction. Literally, he does not know what he needs and such ignorance constitutes a formidable internal barrier to need satisfaction—in short, it is a form of neurosis.

Misdirection

Although the adjusted American remains unfulfilled, he expends incredible amounts of energy attempting to satisfy his needs. Unfortunately, his energy is misdirected. *Misdirection is behavior motivated by a need, but inappropriate to the satisfaction of that need.* To return to the example of the sailor on the raft, this parched fellow may drink salt water in an attempt to satisfy his thirst.

The man who drinks salt water usually does so only in his last extremity, knowing that his behavior is misdirected, probably fatally so. The misdirection which is part of the pattern of normal neurosis, however, is seldom so obvious. Succeeding chapters will detail many such misdirections, but let us consider one example here: the attempt, which takes myriad forms among Americans, to establish an environment which will supposedly make a man happy.

The adjusted American directs much of his energy toward obtaining the accouterments of "the good life," which seems to be the mid-century definition of the pursuit of happiness. But merely occupying the glass-walled house in the suburbs does not guarantee happiness, as a spate of books about suburbanites have amply demonstrated.

Happiness is the emotional state that accompanies need satisfaction. As such, it can be achieved only through action by the individual—it cannot be absorbed by some special osmosis from the environment in which he is placed. A situation is only an *opportunity* to satisfy needs. It is true that the opportunities may be relatively greater in some situations than in others, but the *critical* variable is the effectiveness of the action, not the setting in which it occurs.

The person who holds deprived needs in abeyance while he struggles to set the scene which he expects will bring him happiness is misdirecting his energies, and when he finally settles back to be made happy, he will be sorely disappointed. It is unlikely that he will learn much from the experience, however. He is more likely to doubt his capacity for happiness than to question the means by which he sought it. He feels that by now he *ought* to be happy—he is far enough in debt. Besides, he is convinced that others who have played the same game are happy, and he believes that there must be something wrong with him if he is not. That his neighbors may be concealing a similar disappointment does not seem to occur to him. One is reminded of the emperor's new clothes.

Attempts to create an environment conducive to the satisfaction of needs are not necessarily misdirected. They may be to the point—but only if the focus is kept on meeting needs in the situation. Once creating or maintaining the situation becomes an end in itself, the behavior becomes an example of misdirection, for it will no longer be directed toward satisfying the need which motivated it.

Tension: The Symptom of Need

The third element of normal neurosis involves the misinterpretation of tension. When a person suffers sudden and acute deprivation of a basic need or experiences a threat of such deprivation, he responds with tension. The nervous system triggers certain specific physiological responses: adrenalin pours into the blood stream, the respiratory rate is accelerated, the pulse quickens, blood is diverted from the abdominal viscera to the skeletal muscles, blood pressure rises, extra glucose is released into the blood, and various other bodily responses prepare the organism for immediate and violent action to counter the threat or to overcome the deprivation.

Tension thus serves a function, or is able to do so. The nervous system has responded to deprivation by a surge of available energy with which to meet the emergency. Let us consider an uncomplicated animal response, a sort of parable.[1] Imagine a spring in the hills, surrounded by dense thickets of brambles through which a deer trail winds. A great stag comes toward the spring, but the trail is too narrow for his broad antlers and he is caught in the brambles. The stag hesitates for a moment, adrenalin is released into his blood, his heartbeat and breathing quicken—and with a great surge he tears himself free, charges through the remaining brambles and wades into the spring to drink. The responses of the stag are functional from first to last: moved to action by thirst, he seeks satisfaction; encountering an obstacle, he mobilizes energy, which he utilizes to win through to the water where he slakes his thirst.

The adjusted American, however, has not learned to equate his tension with deprivation. Rather, he tends to interpret his tension as anger, resentment, depression, and the like, which he believes must have some external provocation. Failing to grasp the relation between need and tension, he becomes preoccupied with some supposed cause of his "anger," and neglects the needs which give rise to his tension.

When entangled in obstacles, he regards the resultant tension as anger at the obstacle. He is thus distracted into an attack on whatever manner of brambles surround him, and his surge of energy is misdirected. Had the stag in the parable behaved like the average man, he would have neglected his thirst and turned to uprooting brambles—becoming ever more thristy, more tense ("furious"), more wild in his assault, until he finally collapsed from exhaustion.

There is another common misinterpretation of tension, and another pattern of misdirection that follows from it. To continue the metaphor, if the man caught in the thicket of "brambles" regards his tension as anger at the brambles but is afraid to attack them, he is likely to turn the anger back on himself as depression—to sit down in the thicket and cry. "Mad" thus becomes "sad." But whether the man attacks the brambles or tears his hair, his energy is misdirected. His behavior contributes nothing to the need which led to the mobilization of his energy.

When deprivation is milder but chronic, the bodily responses are less marked but there is nonetheless a state of tension. *Tension is the symptom of needfulness.* The relation of chronic tension to high blood pressure, ulcers, and other visceral disorders has long been established. Normal neurosis, which inhibits the fulfillment of needs and is characterized by chronic tension, is thus a threat to physical as well as mental health.

The interplay of the elements of a normal but neurotic behavior pattern is as follows: a pressing need creates tension which motivates the individual to action; faulty interpretation of the nature of the need leads the individual into misdirected behavior, which leaves him deprived; deprivation, now more extreme, triggers heightened tension; faulty interpretation of this tension (as anger or depression) leads to more frantic but misdirected action—and the squirrel cage whirls around.

3
THE MAINSPRING

The role of both physical and psychological needs in human behavior is strictly that of first causes. Without the spur which they provide, the individual would remain quiescent. RALPH LINTON

Drawing mechanical analogies to human behavior has gone out of fashion, largely because in the past such analogies often implied a rigid determinism in human behavior. Yet, within limits, a mechanical analogy may be useful. Bearing in mind the greater flexibility of human behavior, let us consider the operation of a clockwork mechanism. Such mechanisms differ greatly in what they do—among other things they can meter time, play music boxes, or make dolls dance—but regardless of what the mechanism is doing, it is activated by the pressure of the unwinding mainspring. Any analysis of the mechanism is necessarily an account of the particular way in which this pressure is channeled and manifested.

Similarly, behind all the infinite variety of human behavior lies the pressure of a few basic and universal needs. Whatever men do is a manifestation of these pressures and any analysis of human behavior must begin with them. Needs are the mainspring of human behavior.

In this chapter we shall describe the nature and

origin of the emotional needs which the American struggles to fulfill. In the process we shall be led into a relatively abstract and theoretical discussion. For the professional reader, therefore, this may be the most interesting chapter, since here we provide the theoretical framework for the mode of analysis used throughout the book. For the reader who is unaccustomed to such discussion it may prove the least interesting. We hope, however, that he will consent to wade through it. If he skips or skims this chapter he should nevertheless comprehend what follows, but he will have to take our interpretation of human needs on faith.

Men may satisfy their needs without understanding them; countless generations have eaten when hungry without comprehending body chemistry. But the person who does not understand the nature of his needs is dependent on the traditions of his culture. He will find the fulfillment which normal (that is, customary) behaviors entail, and he will also encounter the deprivations. Thus if eating the normal diet of his culture results in beriberi, he will suffer beriberi; if a sense of personal inadequacy goes along with a normal existence in his culture, he will feel inadequate.

Deprivations which are normal are likely to be tolerated as inevitable. But even the individual who is able to image escaping them is likely to be unable to do so. He will have no reason, for example, to associate the misery of beriberi with the food he eats, and even if he stumbles on the association will have no easy way of planning a more adequate diet.

Anyone who tries to avoid deprivation without first comprehending the nature of his need usually remains closer to conventional behavior than he realizes. He thinks of the usual behavior and then tries to imagine something different, but starting from this point he is apt to end by merely reversing the pattern he is trying to escape. Backing along a cultural rut is even less likely to be rewarding than proceeding forward down it. Even if he somehow climbs out of the rut, he has only blind trial and error to guide him—unless he understands the nature of his need.

Much of the difficulty in comprehending basic needs results from an inherent problem in perception. The individual's awareness of his motivation is not at the level of the basic, underlying need, but is rather of more specific wants: to take a trip, to eat a steak, to win a promotion, to find a sympathetic ear, to seduce a neighbor. Such wants are nearly infinite in number, although the basic needs of which they are merely manifestations are few in number. But unless his cultural heritage includes a formulation of the basic needs, the individual can arrive at them only through a process of abstraction from the detail of his experience.

The abstractions which the individual makes usually employ the traditional assumptions his culture makes regarding human nature, for these are to him the most plausible system of classification. The areas where conventional categories are useful are not, however, the areas of his most pressing deprivation. By and large, those needs which can be perceived clearly in traditional categories are readily satisfied in that cultural milieu. To go beyond normalcy, an individual must come to a better understanding of those basic needs which are generally misunderstood in his culture.

Physical Needs

Whatever else man may be, he is first of all an animal with certain requirements for oxygen, tolerable temperatures, water, sleep, food, and so forth. These needs are so directly vital to life itself that all functioning societies necessarily provide at least minimal fulfillment of them most of the time. Even people existing on a substandard diet must be able to survive long enough to produce the next generation and raise it to puberty, or that society will simply disappear. In contemporary America, the prevailing understanding of the basic physical needs is generally accurate and the cultural patterns provide satisfaction.

There are other needs which have an innate biological basis but which are less essential to the sheer maintenance of life. The needs for muscular, mental, and sexual activity are examples. Because the human organism can tolerate some deprivation in these areas, confusion surrounding them has less obvious consequences than confusion regarding needs more directly related to survival. Perhaps it is not surprising, therefore, that such needs are often subject to cultural misinterpretation.

Thus, to the adjusted American exercise is a word that conjures up images of sweaty people doing push-ups. Yet it has been abundantly demonstrated that a body deteriorates if it is not used, and "fitness" has become a national objective—however oddly it fits with a life style designed for a minimum of physical effort.

Mental activity is equally shunned as disagreeable. Somehow most of the children who enter kindergarten eager to learn emerge from the educational process a dozen years later as young adults who abhor studying. The intellectual stultification of the general populace has been bemoaned by many writers; our point is not just to reiterate that this condition exists, but rather to add that it exists in large measure because most Americans learn not to enjoy exercising their minds.

The normal patterns of American culture are not conducive to uncomplicated satisfaction in using the body and the mind. The normal American adult, therefore, seeks to surround himself with push-button convenience and capsule news. Yet he apparently remains dimly aware of his drive to activity, for he often punishes his children by making them sit still—and not ask questions.

Cultural confusion regarding sexual activity is more complicated, more fraught with tabu and rebellion. Americans generally assume that the sexual behaviors allowed to them are inadequate for full satisfaction. It is often pointed out that Americans are subjected to constant sexual stimulation by the mass media, then left to struggle with a restrictive moral code. In reality, however, there is little evidence that this code leads to much *sexual* deprivation.

For example, monogamy restricts the variety of bed-mates—even making a generous allowance for the prevalence of adultery. Yet the physical need is for sexual activity; variety of partners is irrelevant. A desire for variety is doubtless common, but it derives from other needs which the individual brings with him to the sexual situation (a matter we shall consider in detail in Chapter Eight). George Bernard Shaw summarized the essential point when he said "marriage is popular because it combines the maximum of temptation with the maximum of opportunity." [1] It is difficult to make a case for sexual deprivation among the married!

The unmarried American has no sanctioned sexual outlet, but there is little evidence that this results in deprivation. By all statistics, the unmarried American male has a very high frequency of sexual experience, whether through nocturnal emission, masturbation, homosexual relations, heterosexual relations, or (most probably) a combination of these. Whatever deprivations he suffers are not primarily sexual.

The unmarried American female apparently has less sexual experience than her male counterpart (at least that she is willing to admit), but this hardly establishes that she suffers greater deprivation. A more plausible hypothesis is that the inexperienced female may simply have a more diffuse sexual drive. Americans, married or unmarried, suffer little deprivation which is genuinely sexual.

Most of the problems which the adjusted American experiences in connection with his needs for mental, physical, and sexual activity reflect his profound misunderstandings in yet another area—which we shall term the *self needs*. American culture provides neither a clear understanding of these needs nor adequate customs for satisfying them, and the adjusted American thus experiences both chronic and acute deprivation without really understanding the needs that are being deprived. The anxiety, boredom, and insecurity which are normal in American life are related to the deprivation of self needs much as hunger is related to the need for physical sustenance. The self needs are the crux of normal neurosis in American culture.

The Self Needs

There are certain needs which have no apparent basis in man's physical being but which are, nevertheless, common to all men. The essential universality of such needs was once explained by assuming that they were instinctive; reference was made to supposed instincts of gregariousness, workmanship, self-expression, and the like. This explanation was simple and convenient, but over the years evidence accumulated which indicated that these needs were not instinctive, inborn drives. It has become apparent that the self and the needs associated with it are social in origin, not physical.

From time to time a child is discovered who has been raised in nearly total isolation from other humans. Relegated to an attic or chicken coop, he has somehow survived with the irreducible minimum of attention. When discovered, such a child is human only in the physical sense of the word. He neither speaks nor reasons nor desires companions. He has no sense of identity, no sense of right or wrong, no interest in other people. He lacks, in short, an integrated human personality—a *self*. And, having no self, he has none of the needs for self-expression, self-realization, interaction with other selves, and similar needs that are associated with the human personality.

The near universality of the self needs can be accounted for by the near universality of the basic process of socialization. Men in divergent cultural settings share fundamentally similar experiences in early childhood as they learn to be social beings and in this process certain needs develop which all socialized men share.

There has been considerable study of the process of socialization. Piaget has made extensive contributions to knowledge of how the child constructs reality from perception; George H. Mead and his intellectual heirs have offered profound insights into the development of consciousness of self. Less attention has been directed specifically toward the manner in which the self needs arise as the self is created. Fromm has emphasized that the need for meaningful activity derives from the development of individuation, and Mead, Cooley, and Sartre have all made insightful suggestions on the origins of the need for association. Examples of such contributions could be multiplied, but at this point it seems more important to undertake a systematic analysis of the self needs than to trace the roots from which the analysis derives. The problem can be simply stated: what are the self needs and how do they arise in the process of socialization?

Every human being started at the same point as the isolated child. But in the course of close association with other people he has learned to be human and he has resolved problems with which the isolated child is never confronted. First of all, he has transcended his purely physical existence and developed an awareness of self. This is so easily stated that its profound importance is easily missed. It is this development of self-awareness that differentiates men from the other animals.

The tiny infant has no conception of himself as a person; at the outset he is simply a center where various sensations, pleasant and unpleasant, are experienced. He is not born with a ready-made consciousness of himself. He must acquire, slowly and with great difficulty, an awareness of himself as a being with a continuous existence, endowed with certain capacities and qualities.

The infant begins by differentiating himself from his environment. He must learn the difference between his body and the objects around him. Sometimes finding his thumb in his mouth and sometimes his pacifier, he gradually comes to recognize a consistent difference: he can feel his thumb with his mouth and his mouth with his thumb, but when he sucks his pacifier he has sensation only in his mouth. He learns to distinguish between his sock (which can be detached) and his foot (which cannot). Slowly he learns the physical limits of his body.

At the same time, the child is sorting out internal sensations. The tiny infant may accept food eagerly when he is suffering from colic, but the older baby learns to differentiate the feeling of hunger from that of indigestion and to attach different significance to each. He is learning to interpret his sensations, to understand them as indicating deprivation or satisfaction. He cannot yet say, "I am hungry" or even think it, for he has no words. But he is beginning to have a sense of himself as something which feels, wants, and does.

These initial stages in the development of self-awareness are not uniquely human; thus far the human child proceeds much as a puppy or a kitten. The child has more mental capacity to apply to the task, but the differences are quantitative, not qualitative. It is only when the child begins to learn language that his development takes a qualitatively different turn from that of the young of other complex mammals. In language, the child has the key tool for developing a human self.

As the child learns language, he learns to name the things in the world about him: Mommy, cookie, dog. Having names for these elements of his experience means that he has a symbol which stands for them in his mind. He learns other symbols that describe states of being: nice, naughty, dirty, pretty. With these symbols at his command he can perform complex mental manipulations. Even when his mother is not present he can think about her and in a way that involves more than merely remembering a mental image of how she looks, or feels, or smells. He can link her symbol—her name—experimentally with other symbols: Mommy is pretty, Mommy is dirty, Mommy is a nice boy, Mommy is a dog. By trial combinations of words he learns, he tries to build a symbolic model which will correspond to the Mommy that actually exists.

He learns words that refer to behavior as well as to

things, words such as kiss, go, eat, spank. In terms of these words he can think about how his mother acted yesterday and today, and can attempt generalization: about tomorrow. He establishes the idea of interaction and reciprocity through words such as help and give. By imitation and by trial and error he builds the concepts which enable him to contemplate the world and interpret his experience.

When he learns *his own name* he acquires a momentous tool: a symbol which refers to an abstract entity which both he and others associate with his own being. With this symbol he is able to think about himself, in much the same way that he can think about his mother. (Notice that a small child will *respond* to his name for months before he learns to *speak* it—there seems to be a large mental leap between recognizing that his attention is expected and learning to manipulate the symbol for himself.)

When he learns to use his own name, he begins to perceive a self which has certain characteristics and a continuing existence in time. He notes that others perceive this self, and he struggles to perceive it as they do. He can now try experimentally linking his self symbol with other symbols; he can compare what he was like yesterday with what he is today and can speculate on what he may be tomorrow. He can even talk to himself. As he constructs his *self-image*—a concept which attempts to encompass the totality of his own being—he comes to exist in a conscious and contemplative way that no other animal ever achieves.

This consciousness of self must be learned; it is not innate. Physical characteristics, such as the speech centers of the brain, are essential to it, but maturation of these characteristics is not in itself sufficient to produce the self. Language does not simply erupt at a given age as teeth do; the child raised in isolation gets teeth but not language—nor consciousness of self. The self arises out of socialization, a process of inter-action with other human beings in a world structured by language.

Having become conscious of self, the child loses the unreflective simplicity of the animal. He is irrevocably altered. Barring brain damage or permanent coma, he cannot escape self-awareness once it has developed. *And along with this awareness of self there emerge certain self needs, needs which will hereafter claim an important part of the individual's time and energy.* The development of these needs, common to all so-cialized men, is as irreversible as the consciousness of self.

The needs of the self are closely interrelated, but for analytic clarity we shall separate them into three major aspects: (1) *the need for an accurate and ac-ceptable self-image;* (2) *the need to verify this self-image and expand the self through association;* (3) *the need to verify the self-image and expand the self through action.* Along with the physical needs previ-ously discussed, these self needs constitute the basic needs of man, the driving force behind human be-havior.

The need for an accurate and acceptable self-image. It is useful to distinguish between the self—that which the individual is—and the self-image—his con-ception of what he is. Although the self and the self-image develop together, they are not automatically isomorphic. The self-image is a mental construct and may be a relatively accurate or a relatively inaccurate image of what it symbolizes.

However, if the individual is to act effectively, his conceptions of reality must be approximately accurate reflections of reality. Any inaccurate concept is trou-blesome; it will be acutely so if the concept in question is the most important single concept in the individual's consciousness: his self-image. If his self-image is inaccurate, he will undertake actions which have little chance of success, or conversely (and more commonly) will cut himself off from many things that he could do and enjoy because he has an unrealistically limited self-image. If his self-image is inaccurate, he will feel uncertain and uneasy. Once the self-image is formed, the individual feels a need for it to reflect accurately what he is.

His self-image must also be acceptable—*to himself*. From the very first, the self-image is not neutral, but evaluative. The child builds his image of what he is through his perceptions of what he does. As his actions have consequences which are pleasant or unpleasant, he attaches a corresponding value to the self-potential which they reflect. Those facets of the self which, acted upon, lead to pain (e.g., an urge to play with hot things) he soon assigns a negative value; those facets of the self which, acted upon, lead to pleasure (e.g., the ability to manipulate his spoon) he values positively.

Among the most important consequences of his actions are the responses they elicit from others. We once watched a small boy in a pediatrician's waiting room building a tall tower of blocks. When the tower was finished he deliberately knocked it over with one sweeping blow. As he did so, he chortled, "Good boy!" Then he looked carefully around the room to see how other people (above all his mother) would evaluate his action and what consequences it might have for him.

Most of a child's early self-image is simply a reflection of what others, particularly parents and siblings, tell him he is. These perspectives are at once evaluative and descriptive; he learns how other evaluate him at the same time that he discovers how other perceive him. Told that he is "cute" or "fussy," he learns the built-in evaluation at the same time that he learns the meaning of the term. As he learns to apply words to himself, he applies them both descriptively and normatively. Thus learning to think of himself as a boy is concurrent with learning to think of himself as a good boy, or as a naughty one.

As he internalizes the norms he learns from others, he applies them to himself and wonders if he is acceptable. As he acquires models on which to pattern his devloping self, he accepts standards against which he measures his self-image. It is not so much that he learns to appraise an existing self-image; it would be more accurate to say that his self-image and his evaluation of that image are acquired together. The very idea of being merges with the appraisal of modes of being; the process of self-evaluation is simultaneous with the process of self-discovery. Man needs not only an accurate self-image, but also one that he can accept.

In accordance with his developing judgment of himself, the child's self-image becomes selective. He seeks to develop certain potentialities of the self and to abandon other possibilities. He learns, for instance, that it is not acceptable to be a bully or a "crybaby." He learns of these potentialities as they are pointed out in his own behavior, but he recoils from them and seeks to exclude them from his self-image. Even as he disclaims them, however, he is aware that he could be a bully, that he is trying not to be a "crybaby."

This kind of problem continues throughout the life of the individual. As he matures he inevitably finds a good many elements in himself which clash with the self-image he regards as acceptable. He can deal with this conflict by attempting to make his conception of acceptability one which stresses choice between elements in the self (e.g., "I am capable of being a bully, but I choose not to be"), then acting so as to minimize aspects of the self of which he disapproves. If he succeeds he will be able to satisfy his need for an accurate and acceptable self-image; he will find that he is predominantly acceptable to himself.

Alternatively he may fall into the ineffectual but common attempt to make the self-image acceptable by rendering it inaccurate. This is a basic misdirection, involved in a fundamental—but normal—neurotic pattern. Through a process of self-deceit, the individual may pretend that those aspects of the self of which he disapproves do not exist. The difficulty is that such deception, precisely because it is *self*-deception, inevitably fails. It is because he does perceive in himself elements of which he profoundly disapproves that he seeks to hide these things. In later chapters we shall examine in detail the pitfalls of such attempts at self-deception. Here the essential point is simply that the need of the individual is for a self-image that is *both* accurate and acceptable. Fulfillment does not result if he attempts to sacrifice accuracy for acceptability.

In familiar situations the individual acts in terms of his self-image and his evaluation of that image. In unfamiliar situations he must define and appraise himself in the new context. His self-image is carried forward from situation to situation, but each successive experience leaves its imprint. Throughout his life the individual requires an accurate and acceptable self-image and toward this end he constantly explores, redefines, and evaluates himself. Great novels and dramas have been written about men struggling to know themselves and to accept this knowledge. But as the existentialists have pointed out, the problem is basic and universal in human experience, not confined to the heroic few.

Thus the need which has been variously termed "self-acceptance," "self-understanding," "self-love," and the like is neither innate nor obscure in nature and origin. It is essentially a need for an image of the self which is accurate enough to be workable and acceptable enough so that the individual can enjoy experiencing and expressing it. He needs to feel that he can accept an accurate image of himself and that the image he accepts is accurate. The need is an inevitable by-product of learning to be a social being and emerges with the developing awareness of self. Only by fulfilling it can the human being find inner peace and fulfillment. This is not the unreflective fulfillment of the animal, but a functional equivalent of it at a more complex level of consciousness.

The need to verify the self-image and expand the self through association. The human need for association with others is a matter of universal experience, although the precise nature and origin of this need are often subject to confusion. Viewed as an aspect of the self needs, however, the need for association assumes its logical role in a functionally related whole.

The self-image can never be established once and for all; if it is to be accurate, it must reflect the self as it exists in the present. Although drawn out of past experience, it must accurately mirror what the individual is *now*. Verifying and expressing a self-image which he values is a source of deep satisfaction for the individual. Moreover, by expanding the self in ways consistent with his desired self-image he opens new areas for the fulfillment of his self needs. Association with other people is one of the major means of achieving these ends.

First of all, man requires association as a means of

self-discovery. In childhood he learns to think of himself first through the categories others apply to him. As he struggles to develop his self-image, his parents and later his playmates offer him perspectives of himself as viewed from the outside. He seeks to see himself as others see him and soon he begins trying to imagine how he would appear to a "generalized other," in George Herbert Mead's phrase. By the time he is an adult he finds it difficult to think about himself apart from the way he imagines others perceive him. Even when he is alone, he has a sense of how he would appear to an observer.

The adult remains concerned with the way others perceive him even if he is relatively indifferent to whether or not they like him. (Indeed, his self-image may require being disliked by certain people.) Imagining how he appears when viewed as he can never view himself—as an external object—and verifying this conception of himself through the response he elicits from others remains an invaluable means of self-examination throughout his life. In validating and expanding the perception of the self by the self, the individual requires association with others. *They are his mirrors.*

Secondly, he needs association with others to see what *they* are, and, by extension, what he might be. As he shapes himself, the characteristics of others are valuable points of reference. From them he acquires a conception of the range of human behavior, a kaleidoscopic view of the possibilities of being. Consciously or unconsciously, he imitates those characteristics which appeal to him, discovering new capacities within himself. This process is most marked in childhood, but it continues throughout the life of the individual. He also recognizes in others potentialities which he wishes to avoid in himself. He enlarges his view of his own potential through observing others. *They are his models.*

Finally, but by no means least in importance, association with other people provides the only possible situation in which the individual can experience many aspects of the self. Having been raised in association with other people, he finds that much of his self-image involves interpersonal relationships. He may picture himself as proud, friendly, aloof, sympathetic, forgiving, vindictive, but in order to *be* any of these things he must interact with someone else. He can be neither kind nor cruel in solitude. Because many of the most basic components of the self require the presence of others, the individual's continuing need to verify his self-image and to experience valued aspects of the self impels him to seek association with others. *They are the recipients of his actions.*

Men who are deprived of association for long periods of time usually try to alleviate their deprivation by investing their surroundings with synthetic personalities. The proverbial prospector and his mule are a good case in point. By interacting with his mule as if it were human, the lonely prospector was able to experience many aspects of himself which could not be called forth in solitude. By endowing the mule with a personality quite different from his own, he tried to make the animal useful as a contrasting model. By pretending that the mule discussed and described his actions at length, the prospector tried to make of the animal a mirror. Prisoners in extended solitary confinement have been known to play the same game with spiders.

Paradoxical though it may seem, it is when the individual is with others that he is best able to enjoy and expand many aspects of himself, to refine and verify his self-image. But what has not been said may be as important to an understanding of the need for association as what we have said. Nothing here supports the common assumption that people have a need for the love or admiration of others. Rather, as will be shown in later chapters, the desire for these responses derives largely from lack of self-acceptance. Other people are essential to the individual as mirrors, models, and the recipients of his actions, but their acceptance of him is not a substitute for self-acceptance.

The need to verify the self-image and expand the self through action. The need for activity which is physically based can be satisfied by random action, but self needs lead the individual to seek purposeful action as a means of experiencing, exploring, and expanding his capacities. The process is most obvious in the small child as he experiments continuously with his capabilities. He wants to try whatever he sees others doing and passes through a stage when his response to most situations is "Me do!" The child takes delight in newly discovered abilities, repeating over and over again some new sound he has learned to make, mashing his cookie in order to pick up each crumb, taking off his shoe as often as his mother is willing to put it back on his foot. Developing a self is an active process.

The same process can be observed in the adolescent as he matches himself against his environment, trying his capabilities, seeking the limits of the self. The American boy buys a car to see if he can make it run, and, having made it run, risks his life to see what he can make it do. In dozens of similar experiments, he acquires an expanding sense of what he is through the things he does. A boy becoming a man, he seeks to discover what manner of man he may be.

Similarly, the adolescent girls tests her capacities. She tries on theatrical mannerisms, conforms passionately to the shifting customs of her clique, and experiments with her femininity. Intensely aware that she is becoming a woman, she is preoccupied with testing her appeal to boys, seeking to see how she measures up to her image of a desirable woman. Testing the self to see what one may be becoming plays a central role in the frantic pace and volatile emotional experience of the American adolescent. Popular speech reflects this, explaining the actions of youth with such observations as "He is unsure of himself," or "He hasn't found himself yet."

In *The Red Badge of Courage*, Stephen Crane builds a classic novel around the quest of a young soldier for knowledge of himself. The raw recruit is preoccupied with the question of how he will act under fire. Will he run? Through agonizing months of waiting for battle, he torments himself with this question—but he knows that he can never be sure he is not a coward until he faces the situation he dreads, not so much for its inherent danger as for the self-revelation that he may find there.

Even in mundane situations, the individual must *act* in order to discover what he is, and he must act in order to conutinue experiencing aspects of himself which he values and enjoys. If he thinks of himself as a businessman, a parent, an athlete, an intellectual, he must engage in behavior appropriate to this self-image. If he does not, he must redefine himself, or he will be left anxious and needful. (Here is the reason for the psychological shock of retirement; the man who has retired may find that suddenly he can no longer *be* that which he most valued himself for being.)

Past actions through which he sought to know and to accept the self are not capable of satisfying this need in the present. Recalling the past can only remind the individual of what he used to be. The erstwhile football hero who is still reliving the big game fifteen years later, or the ex-campus queen who tries to give meaning to her life by clinging to her reign over the prom of a decade ago, are pathetic figures. As the existentialists have pointed out, man must act in order to be, and what he becomes is largely the summation of his actions.

In any situation, at any given moment, a man chooses his actions. The difference between adjustment and autonomy is not whether the individual is able to choose, for choose he must. The issue is rather whether he makes choices consciously or by default. The adjusted individual is largely unaware of choosing his actions; the person capable of choosing autonomously has a heightened awareness of choice and of its implications for himself and for his self-acceptance.

The adjusted American has learned to regard his personality as an expression of what he was born to be, or what he was conditioned to be, and to assume that he can never change dramatically (except, perhaps, for the worse). There are many people who cling to this conception of a determined self because they shrink from accepting responsibility for being what they are. Those who cannot accept themselves find a false comfort in believing that heredity, society, parents, or whatever, is responsible for the shaping of their lives. For such solace as this belief affords them, they trade the possibility of choosing their lives differently and creating a more acceptable self.

To be sure, those who surround the individual during early childhood greatly influence his initial conception of himself and the type of choices he learns to make. But he is not molded irrevocably by the age of four or five. A man is more than the synopsis of his childhood—or at least he can be more. The self is never rigidly defined until the moment of death; it changes subtly with every choice of action the individual makes. In action piled on action, he becomes a certain kind of person and in a real sense continuously creates himself. He can, if he has sufficient understanding, create a self which he can enjoy.

In summary, three basic needs underlie the complex psychological strivings of the individual: the need for an accurate and acceptable self-image, and the related needs to validate the self-image and to experience and expand the self through association and through action. These three needs are closely interrelated; in fact they can be separated only analytically. Through actions in association with others, the individual develops a self and forms a self-image. This self-image can be found acceptable only if he has confidence that it accurately reflects the self, and such verification is established through further action and association. The process cannot be short-circuited by self-deception; manipulations of the self-image which are not verified through action and association leave the individual with the fear that his self-image is a fraud and that lurking behind it is an unacceptable self.

Few would challenge that these needs exist; what may be more controversial is our contention that these three needs alone account for the nonorganic element of human motivation. Such a contention requires justification and we shall attempt to provide it in the following chapters by showing how human behavior can be understood without positing any further basic needs.

4
MIRROR OF HATRED

That hatred springs more from self-contempt than from a legitimate grievance is seen in the intimate connection between hatred and a guilty conscience.

ERIC HOFFER

In the Middle East of antiquity it was the custom to hold a ceremony from time to time in which the village priest cast evil spirits out of the people and into a goat. Having invested the goat with their own evil, the people fell upon it with sticks and drove it from the village. As the currency of the term *scapegoat* suggests, the practice has persisted over the centuries —but men, not goats, now serve as porters for the disowned sins of others.

Men hate in others those things—and only those things—which they despise in themselves. It is possible to disapprove of other people in a rational and dispassionate manner, but to hate them is an irrational and impassioned act. The passion betrays the underlying self-contempt. Hatred is a barrier to self-acceptance. Hatred is a normal neurosis.

The origin of hatred lies in the individual's attempt to disown certain potentialities of the self. It is not possible to expurgate unwanted capacities from the self by denying that they exist. Yet it is normal to try to do so, to attempt to achieve self-acceptance through

41

a process of self-deceit which we shall term *alienation*. *Alienation is the failure to acknowledge aspects of the self, which are then seen as alien.* The person remains aware of his disowned capacities—they do not cease to exist—but he rationalizes his awareness of them by contending that they belong to someone else. He *projects* his alienated characteristics onto any convenient bystander, where he can view them with indignation and contempt. As we shall use the term, a *projection* is an alienated aspect of the self which is attributed to someone else.

Hating Collectively

It may become a general custom to alienate certain self-potential and to project it onto a particular group of people—the scapegoats of a society. The sum of such projections constitutes the *stereotype* of this despised group. Such stereotypes are defended ardently against all evidence which contradicts them. These irrational and impassioned steretotypes underlie the collective hatred which is termed, somewhat euphemistically, prejudice. Prejudice is found to some degree in all adjusted Americans. The fanatic racist merely carries the pattern farther than is normal.

The racist who insists that integration must be resisted, by violence if necessary, justifies his position on the grounds that Negroes are too dirty, stupid, lazy, irresponsible, and promiscuous to mingle with whites. The fascinating aspect of the stereotype is that it represents the values of the American middle class turned inside out; that is to say, it embodies the rejected—and alienated—potential of the middle-class American.

The middle-class child is taught that he must be clean, bright, ambitious, and chaste. He may harbor a longing to be unwashed, indolent, carefree, and sensual, but he learns to alienate such desires and to project them onto ethnic minorities, especially onto Negroes (in some parts of the Southwest, Mexicans may be the target for such projections). If his emotions surrounding his alienated potential are mild, he is normal. If his feeling is intense, he may grow up to be a fanatic racist.

Projecting his own fascination with sex, the racist contends that Negroes are sensual and promiscuous. The projection of his own desire to avoid responsibility leads to his assertion that Negroes are shiftless, unable to manage their own affairs, require and actually welcome paternalistic domination. (He sees nothing contradictory in his further assertion that Negroes do not need higher wages because they are able to "get along" on less money than whites—which surely implies either a superior capacity to manage money or ascetic self-denial.) Feeling uneasy about his own dishonesty (petty or otherwise), he points accusingly at Negroes (or Puerto Ricans, or Mexicans), as untrustworthy thieves.

The racist argues that Negroes fit the stereotype. If this were universally true it would not alter the fact that the racist is projecting. His passion betrays a recoiling from alienated sides of himself. Moreover, it is interesting to note that considerable effort is expended by racists (and not only in the South) to force the Negro to fit the stereotype. In *Black Boy*, Richard Wright vividly portrayed his struggle to pretend that he was what his white bosses expected him to be: stupid, dishonest, and carefree.

The racist uses Negroes as a depository for his projections, and it would be painful to him to abandon the stereotype which justifies his projections. For this reason, he responds with bewildered fury to the Negro professor, lawyer, engineer, or physician. By careful conformance to middle-class values, the Negro professional threatens the stereotype. (A Negro college president reports being seated next to a white woman at a luncheon; she could apparently think of nothing to say to him, but finally blurted out, "Don't you just love watermelon?")

If the scapegoat minority group is so useful a target for projections, why is it (symbolically at least) driven out of the village? Aggression against minority groups is an attempt to destroy the despised projections hung on them, or at least to drive them to a safe distance. (It should be noted that most members of such a group are seldom driven farther than the outskirts of town.)

There are other motives for aggression against a scapegoat minority. Often such a group is a convenient substitute for a powerful group that people are afraid to attack. The fact that lynchings in the South used to become more frequent when the price of cotton dropped is an excellent illustration of such displaced aggression. The people who controlled the cotton market were remote and/or powerful; the Negroes were handy and helpless. Political and religious minorities as well as racial minorities often serve as targets for displaced aggression—hence the affinity between racists and far-right hate groups.

Aggression against a minority group leads to more intense hatred of that group. As Eric Hoffer points out, man hates those he has wronged and only rarely those who have wronged him. Underlying this curious twist in human behavior is the simple fact that few people can see themselves as cruel without violating their self-image. When a man does something which violates his self-image he experiences guilt: that is, self-loathing. The only way to ease guilt is through action which brings the self-image back to something the individual can accept. But often the guilt-laden person seeks to justify his behavior rather than to amend it. If the victim of cruelty is cast as a villain himself, then the cruelty can be rationalized as retribution. And thus it is that he who has been injured may be able to forgive, but the person who inflicted the injury hates his victim with rising passion.

The adjusted American wants to be fair, and discrimination against minorities contradicts his idea of equal opportunity for all. He is uneasy if he perceives that he is himself taking advantage of some group through the cheap labor he hires or the special privilege he enjoys because others are excluded. Such guilty discomfort exists even among white Southerners who have been taught from childhood that special privilege is their due. They have all learned the American ideal of equal opportunity and the Christian ideal of brotherhood and they experience an uneasy ambivalence, a pervasive sense of guilt.

The racist transmutes his guilt into hatred. He justifies his actions by citing the depravity of the Negro: that is, by pointing to the projections he has hung on the Negro. The effect of this is a vast increase in the racist's emotional stake in maintaining the projections of which his prejudice is compounded. It is usually assumed that prejudice is the cause of discrimination. The converse is at least equally true. Those who discriminate experience a guilt which creates a vested interest in preserving prejudice. *So long as discrimination exists, people will cling to prejudice.*

In his desire to maintain his prejudice, the racist finds that he is threatened by that facet of himself which regards segregation as unfair. He alienates such feelings, projects them where they seem to fit and then responds with further hatred. He finds the local high school a hotbed of integrationist sentiment and demands a purging of faculty and library. He advocates ruthless treatment of those who espouse civil rights. But the demand for justice which rankles most cannot be purged, for it wells up within himself. The New Orleans mother with child on hip, shrieking obscenities at children entering a newly integrated school, flung her curses at her own sense of guilt.

The Hatred of Hatred

Although many Americans despise prejudice, none escapes it. The liberal's mother may have taught him that all men are created equal, but his aunt may have scolded, "Don't put that penny in your mouth—you don't know what nigger might have had it in his pocket!" From the children on his block he learns, "Eenie, meenie, minie, moe, catch a nigger by the toe. . . ." Or perhaps he learns as standard usage that to bargain sharply is "to Jew down." If not from his family, then from his playmates, or from echoes of the larger society, the American child becomes acquainted with prejudice and to some degree learns to respond in a prejudiced way to customary scapegoats.

As an adult, he may rationally reject stereotypes as fallacious and emotionally recoil from bigotry. Yet his streak of prejudice exists as one aspect of ambivalent feelings. If he can learn to recognize and accept the prejudiced side of his nature, he can also recognize that it is an insignificant counterpart to his belief in equality, a residue of feeling that need not interfere with his actions nor threaten his self-image as a liberal. But if he is unwilling to admit his vestigial prejudice, it will bother him.

Picture a dedicated integrationist eating in a restaurant. A Negro couple enter and sit at the next table. The integrationist has an ambivalent response to the Negroes: on the one hand, he is conscious of being pleased with the chance to implement convictions dear to his self-image, a feeling he acts on by nodding in a friendly fashion to the Negro man as their eyes meet. But at the same time he has a faint desire to put the Negroes down. He cannot admit to such a feeling, so he alienates it and looks around to see who the bigot may be. He needs to find at least one.

A man and his wife are preparing to leave a nearby table. Most of her pie is still on her plate and he has not finished his coffee; the uneasy integrationist seizes on these observations as evidence that this couple is departing in a prejudiced huff. He denounces them to his dinner companions and feels a reassuring surge of righteous indignation.

It is possible that the couple did leave because of racial prejudice; it is also possible that they had finished their dinner. In either case, the integrationist is projecting. The feelings of which he is so aware are necessarily his own—there is no way to experience the feelings of anyone else.

Had there not been a couple leaving, he would have found another target for his alienated prejudice. Perhaps the waiter was slow in reaching the Negroes' table; this could have been seized on as evidence that the waiter was the bigot. Anyone speaking with an inflection that revealed Southern origins would have been a handy depository for the alienated prejudice. (And here this liberal would have slipped into the same process of stereotyping he deplores.) The point is that he would have found someone who seemed a likely target for his projected prejudice. Starting with the conviction that he knew how *someone* was feeling, he had only to pick a candidate.

The integrationist who cannot acknowledge his own streak of prejudice (and there are many who do learn to accept and live with this facet of themselves) is caught up in a futile attempt to eradicate a part of himself. Projection distorts his view of himself and of others and interferes with his efforts to promote civil rights. He is not free to deal with people objectively or to recognize and tap the sense of justice in people who are indeed more prejudiced than he. He usually succeeds only in antagonizing people whom he "discovers" to be prejudiced and seeks to purify.

If someday he learned to accept the fact that he was himself capable of prejudice, he could place his feelings in proper perspective. After an initial period of uneasiness, he would find that he was mostly unbiased with just a conventional residue of bigotry. His prejudice would no longer frighten him, for having accepted its existence he could subordinate it to the stronger side of his ambivalence, his belief in equality.

The hatred which we call prejudice and the hatred of this hatred arise from the same misdirection: the attempt to make the self-image acceptable by making it inaccurate. That such individual neurosis has social consequences is abundantly evident in the racial discrimination and violence that characterize our society.

Preaching among the Heathen

However antithetical to the desired self-image, unwanted potential remains in the self and forms the basis of an inevitable ambivalence. The adjusted American recognizes the possibility of ambivalence, but not its inevitability. He has learned to regard conflicting desires and contradictory beliefs as the mark of a vacillating or weak-willed man, and he feels uncomfortable when he becomes aware of his own mixed feelings. Moreover, he tends to regard ambivalence as a temporary state of confusion which will pass as soon as he makes up his mind. Yet only under unusual circumstances can he have anything but ambivalent feelings.

A person is unambivalent only with regard to those few beliefs, attitudes, and characteristics which are truly universal in his experience. Thus a man might believe that the world is flat without really being aware that he did so—if everyone in his society shared this assumption. The flatness of the world would be simply a "self-evident" fact.

But if he once became *conscious* of thinking that the world is flat, he would be capable of conceiving that it might be otherwise. He might then be spurned to invent elaborate proofs of its flatness, but he would have lost the innocence of absolute and unambivalent belief. Being conscious of a belief inspires a certain skepticism, for the person who is aware of believing can also imagine *not* believing. He does not necessarily abandon the conviction; on the contrary, it may come to dominate his thought and action. However, antithetical possibilities flit through his mind.

Conversely, the person who vehemently disbelieves is quite aware of the possibility of believing. Even those ideas that a man never learns to take seriously are nonetheless within the scope of his potential belief. Merely having a name for something—witches, say, or flying saucers—seems to establish a certain credence in it, however much the dominant attitudes of the individual may negate its possibility.

No rejected belief is ever completely discredited. What has once been believed lingers on as a faint possibility. There were once an atheist and a Christian who spend endless hours arguing about religion. Each man felt morally indignant about the other's religious convictions and hoped to bring him to the Truth. One of these men had grown up in a highly religious family, but rebelling during his teens had read the works of the great skeptics, studied the philosophical problems of theology, and become a convinced atheist. The other man had a curiously similar, though opposite, background. Reared by skeptical parents, he too had rebelled, but his rebellion carried him toward religion. He became a devout and singularly well-informed Christian, capable of discussing the great religious thinkers from Augustine to Kierkegaard.

These two men argued almost daily; to each the conversion of the other had become a major goal. Each expressed surprise that anyone as clever as the other could hold such mistaken beliefs. One would point out an absurdity in the position of the other, only to be met with a searching question concerning his own assumptions. Yet in all their thought about the isues of religion, neither ever asked the crucial question about himself: why was he so anxious to convert the other?

Each had started life with one set of beliefs and later had altered his self-image to incorporate an opposing set. But a childhood belief does not disappear merely because the adult decides it is invalid. The adult conviction dominates the stage but the belief of childhood lingers in the wings.

Being free of religious belief was a major element in the self-image of the atheist and the remnants of his childhood faith galled him. He therefore alienated them and projected them onto the Christian. His attack on the latter's religious convictions was an attempt to expurgate a facet of himself. In the curious illogic of misdirection, it seemed that his own self-image would be strengthened if the Christian would renounce his religion.

This Christian was caught up in a parallel but opposite inner debate. His religious beliefs were central to his self-image, and he felt it was terribly important to be able to believe totally and without reservation. Yet his conversion could not eradicate all traces of his childhood among skeptics. The doubts which crossed his mind disturbed him, and he projected them onto the atheist. In seeking to convert the latter, he was first of all seeking to silence the skeptic within.

Both men were engaged in a futile argument. In the unlikely event that one were successful in persuading the other to change his beliefs, neither would find peace. The victor would not have altered his own ambivalence by converting his antagonist and he would need to find another target for his projections. The vanquished would merely have submerged the formerly dominant aspect of his ambivalent beliefs, alienating one side as he embraced the other. It is likely that the pair (whether as two atheists or as two Christians) would have sought out a third man from the opposing camp, projected their now similar alienated beliefs onto him, and sought his conversion. Each was doomed to endless and sterile argument— with himself.

However, if either came to recognize that he was arguing with a disowned facet of himself, he could escape the futile debate. Once he acknowledged the existence of his vestigial beliefs, he could perceive their essential unimportance. He might continue to discuss religious questions, but it would no longer be because he was trying to dispel inner doubts. Rather, it would be because he enjoyed discussing beliefs which were important to him.

The fanatic who refuses to admit the existence of a feared facet of himself may eventually be confronted with undeniable evidence that he harbors the very attitudes or desires he has sought to eradicate in others. The shock may destroy him. A literary case in point is Somerset Maugham's "Rain": self-recognition is sudden and shattering for the missionary who has tried to reform the prostitute, Sadie Thompson.

In general, attempts to convert, reform, or discredit others because their views are despicable reflect an alienated (and despised) sympathy with the views in question. This is true even when the individual is vaguely aware of his own ambivalence. If he responds with righteous indignation to the viewpoint in others, it is because he is unable to fully accept its counterpart in himself.

The Devil Within

Ambivalence is as inevitable in behavior as in belief. Every way of being and acting has antithetical alternatives, and to be conscious of one is to be conscious of the other. The inherent logic of English (and other Indo-European languages) promotes this by providing logical opposites: a word such as *kind* is meaningless without the antithetical concept, *unkind*. In order to think of himself as kind, a person must be aware of what he would do if he were unkind. Indeed, he expresses his kindness as much by abstaining from cruel acts as by performing kind ones. He is necessarily aware of his capacity to be either kind or cruel, but he does not necessarily permit himself to be aware of his desire to be both.

The fact that certain behaviors are tabu does not mean that people have no desire to engage in them; Pandora and Eve are universal symbols. As a "do not open" sign piques curiosity, so all forbidden behaviors acquire a special fascination. Moreover, people who are pointed to as horrible examples often appear to be enjoying themselves immensely and even people who pride themselves on moral purity may suspect that certain behaviors are forbidden because they are fun. Most children find that it is precisely when they are most enjoying themselves that their mothers call, "Stop that instantly!"

The fear of punishment or ostracism is usually great enough to prevent most people from indulging in forbidden behavior (when most do indulge, the behavior usually ceases to be forbidden). In addition to virtue founded on fear, there is abstention based on the self-image. Most people have learned to want to be the kind of person who behaves according to the ethic of his society. Thus, to break the tabus is to violate the self-image.

And thus it is that the individual is both drawn to and repelled by forbidden behavior. Even though he never quite dares to try it, even though his desire to abstain is overwhelmingly stronger, the faint contradictory desire remains. Ambivalence is universal and inevitable; the self is not a harmonious set of characteristics but rather an intricate balance of contradictions.

This is not to say that the pull of both desires is always equally strong. In general a person will have incorporated one side of the ambivalence into his self-image, and he is more highly motivated to act in accordance with his self-image than to explore his capacity to violate it. Were no other problems involved, he could act on the stronger of his desires or beliefs as a means of expressing and experiencing the self-image he wants to maintain. Contradictory desires would simply be overruled.

But people often seek to conceal one aspect of their ambivalence, particularly when they have learned to regard it as wrong to have such a desire. One of the misguided assumptions of American culture is the notion that an acceptable person does not have unacceptable desires. That this conviction is unrealistic offers not the slightest deterrent to its persistence in the culture; each person simply remains uncomfortable with his secret thoughts. He never realizes, for example, that the truly compassionate man is one who recognizes and overrules minor sadistic inclinations.

Believing that to feel a forbidden desire is morally equivalent to acting on it, the adjust American is afraid to admit that he has such desires. If he hesitantly confesses awareness of his potential desire to act in ways he considers dishonest, sadistic, or depraved, other people (concealing similar desires) respond with alarm. He soon arrives at some appalling self-doubts and a sense of moral weakness that he strives to hide from others—and from himself. At this point he alienates the forbidden desire.

The pretense that a facet of the self does not exist makes its persistence a guilty secret. An alienated characteristic thus assumes an importance far out of proportion to its relative weight in the person's ambivalent feelings. Projected onto someone else, it becomes monstrous.

And herein lies the genesis of hatred. Having projected alienated self-potential onto another, the individual sees in this person only the magnified reflection of despised parts of himself. This means that he sees the other as wholly despicable and himself as the very model of virtue. He wants to destroy this person who is the epitome of evil—not recognizing that what he wants to destroy is the projected image of himself *as he imagines and fears he might be.*

When Hanging Is Too Good

A young tough stamps an old woman to death. Shock and rage sweep the city, and the murdered becomes an object of mass hatred. Some people lament the passing of the whipping post, and others shout for the death penalty. One should like to think old women could walk without fear, and to believe youths incapable of such assaults. But why does the murderer evoke such intense hatred? Why the impassioned cry for his destruction? Why do people come from all over the city to see the spot where the old woman fell, to look for drops of blood on the wall of a building?

Logic suggests the answer: there lurks within each breast a small and secret desire to murder, rape, and pillage. How else can the general fascination with crimes of violence be understood? How else explain the fact that every notorious killer becomes a national hero in disguise, every murder trial an absorbing public event?

Because the adjusted individual experiences the deprivations which are normal in his society, he experiences the tension which reflects chronic deprivation. This tension is interpreted as anger, with the result that he feels a continuous sense of rage, varying from mild annoyance to fury. *Needfulness is thus transmuted to rage—and then to outrage.* The individual assumes that he has been provoked by those who seem to block his desires: first his parents, later his teachers, ultimately authority in general. There is a part of every man that longs to strike out at that ultimate thicket of brambles, society itself. Smash—burn—destroy—and any group or individual can serve as a symbol for the whole.

Yet to admit such violent desires seems threatening, and the adjusted person alienates this potential. But alienation cannot excise it from the self. The capacity for brutality is still experienced, and the sensational crime is exciting because it titillates the average man's own latent sadism. If he perceives even dimly why he is so fascinated by violence, he is likely to recoil in horror from the perception.

The presence of the criminal offers a convenient

opportunity for projection. The adjusted man can assert that it is the murderer who has aroused his horror. He demands the killer's death, claiming to know that the youth will never change, that his vicious nature will represent a threat to society as long as he is allowed to live. Perhaps, but it is the potential murderer within that he sees so clearly, and though the offender be sent to the gas chamber or to prison for life, the man who demands his destruction remains unchanged. The frightening side of the solid citizen remains. Aware that *someone* is contemplating unspeakable horrors, he searches the newspaper for him.

Beyond Hatred

The accusations which A hurls at B are embarrassing bits of A's autobiography. The insights which A has into B's sick motivations reveal the motives of A, for one person can have insight into another only by analogy to his own experience. Whether or not the projections fit, the accusations and the insights are best applied where they originate—within the self.

Like all other misdirections, hatred and righteous indignation consume energy without leading to the fulfillment of the need which is motivating the individual. They are misdirected responses to the need for an accurate and acceptable self-image; the individual seeks to make his self-image acceptable by falsifying it. Such self-deception can never succeed fully, for a subliminal awareness of the hidden desire is inevitable. This awareness leads to defensiveness about the projection, to indignant denials of the true nature of the projection, to attacks on the "hated" others. When hatred is translated into assaults on others, guilt mounts, the need to find the self acceptable increases alarmingly, and so does the tension which accompanies need. The individual interprets this increased tension as rising anger, or mounting hatred, and thus the misdirection feeds itself. He who hates is unfree, and consumed by a neurotic passion.

To become autonomous, it is necessary to move beyond hatred. Yet, when a person first senses that what he despises in others is a mirrored image of latent potential in himself, he is fearful. It seems that if he looked closely he would discover that he was the antithesis of all that he hoped to be. A hitherto unconcealed aspect of the self does loom large at the moment of recognition, but once it becomes familiar it slips into place in the totality of the self. Only the man who can honestly admit that "nothing human is alien to me" is capable of self-acceptance.

Hatred is not natural, it is only a normal neurosis. It is normal to fail to recognize the frightening aspects of the self, to alienate and project them, and then to despise them in others. It is for this reason that hatred fails to excite the wonder of the adjusted American. He takes it for granted that it is natural to hate and he loses thereby the opportunity to understand his emotional experience and to deal with it.

As long as the internal conflict persists unrecognized, the hated others are indispensable to the very people who hate them. Those who hate require a target for their projections, and if a plausible target does not exist they will invent one. There could have been no medieval mind without Satan, Nazi Germany depended on its dwindling supply of Jews, the Chinese utilize the war-mongering imperialists, and the Birch Society must find its Communists.

5
THE PERSECUTED

. . . he was defeated long before he died because, at the bottom of his heart, he really believed what white people said about him. . . . You can only be destroyed by believing that you really are what the white world calls a nigger. JAMES BALDWIN

Whereas the person who projects frightening aspects of himself onto others sees the world filled with evil which he wants to destroy, the person who projects self-condemnation sees a world filled with people who want to destroy him. The first is prone to feeling righteously indignant, the second to feeling persecuted.

Second-Class Citizen
The member of a subordinated minority encounters hostility and discrimination which have nothing to do with him as an individual. He is inescapably encumbered with the projections which form the stereotype of his group. His cultural adaptation requires sensitivity to the shade of meaning in a remark or a gesture, for particularly if discrimination is covert he must learn to respond to subtle cues. Unlike the McWASP (Middle-class-White-Anglo-Saxon Protestant), the member of a subordinated minority learns to look for hostile intent in the trivial disappoint-

ments and snubs of daily life. A low grade, a traffic summons, a slow waiter, an indifferent salesgirl, an unsuccesful job application, inevitably raise for him the question of discrimination. Persecuted for reasons beyond his control, it is easy for him to feel hopelessly trapped. It may be instructive to take this extreme case, where there is objective persecution, to illustrate how projected self-contempt may seem to be hostility from others.

The member of a subordinated minority is often the product of a deprived home environment and is likely to have more than the usual number of problems, neuroses, and misdirections to imitate. Quite as debilitating is the fact that from the earliest awareness of self he has perceived his ethnic identity as his most salient characteristic. The world has not allowed him to ignore it. Constantly reminded that he is a Negro, a Jew, a Mexican, a Puerto Rican, or whatever his group may be labeled, the member of a subordinated minority has almost inevitably made his ethnic identity the core of his self-image. In most associations he has had with the majority he has been subtly—or crudely—reminded that he is expected to personify a stereotype. The cultural milieu in which he was born and reared has pressed on him scorned qualities and insisted that he be contemptible.

In effect, this means that his culture not only has failed to provide him with a useful pattern for finding satisfaction of his self needs, but indeed has gone so far as to insist that he be deprived of the fulfillment of his basic need for an acceptable self-image. To turn the discussion specifically to the most profound minority group struggle in America of the 1960's, the American Negro is perhaps above all involved in a struggle to win the right to view himself without contempt.

The first barrier is the depth to which the prejudiced attitudes of the majority are likely to have penetrated the thinking of the Negro himself. A Negro intellectual, commenting on the movie *Ben-Hur*, remarked, "Just like in a Western, the bad guy had the black horse and the white guy had the good horse." He failed to notice the "accidental" transposition of words which reflected an unconscious equation of white with good.

It is not out of evil caprice that Black Nationalist groups have inverted such values and insisted that black is good, white is evil. It is often easier to invert a pattern than to transcend it. Thus the Black Muslims portray the white man as depraved, dishonest, promiscuous, concerned only with things of the flesh. Like all other attempts to find self-acceptance by projecting feared and despised potential onto others, this attempt is misdirected and neurotic. But it reflects the Negroes' aching need to escape the self-image the culture has imposed on them.

Thus the minority group member typically experiences chronic and acute deprivation of his need for an accurate acceptable self-image, and his level of tension is correspondingly high. As we have observed before, in American culture the tension which accompanies deprivation is usually interpreted as anger—and a desire to strike out at the supposed cause of the "anger." Being unusually vulnerable to reprisal, the minority group member is acutely uncomfortable with his inner rage. He believes that if he were to express it he would be crushed by a world already set against him. He would like to purge himself of his endemic anger, but, because this "anger" is fundamentally needfulness, he is unable to dispel it.

Typically, therefore, he seeks to rid himself of his chronic rage through alienating and projecting it onto others—that is, by seeing it as other people's anger. His projection is made quite plausible by the hostility he does encounter. Adding his own projected anger to the hostility that others do direct toward him, he finds the world a hostile place indeed!

The generalized hostility that he projects is augmented by other, more specific, projections. Unable to find himself acceptable he seeks as a minimum to reduce his feelings of self-contempt by projecting them onto others. To the prejudice of others, which he might learn to take in stride, he adds the frightening reflection of his own self-contempt. Such a man sees hostility and contempt everywhere, for he projects both. He can easily become preoccupied with trying to counteract, or escape, the animosity in which he feels enveloped.

He may respond with thinly veiled aggression. Such behavior invites further hostility, for others find him a convenient target for further negative projections. A vicious circle is set in motion in which about the only compensation is a ready-made rationalization for all his difficulties. If he loses a job or a friend, he can contend that the reason was his refusal to be merely submissive. This rationalization, however, only reinforces his projections of hostility and prejudice.

If he is somewhat more sophisticated, he may cloak his war with the world in ideological trappings and throw himself into the struggle for equality. But the struggle for civil rights requires different tactics from a one-man assault on the social order, and a hostile, aggressive man is likely to become a liability to the cause he espouses.

Many invert the pattern. Imitating the behavior of the prejudiced McWASP, they alienate their self-contempt and become prejudiced themselves. In extreme cases they may try to disassociate themselves from their ethnic group and to pass as McWASPS, or a reasonable facsimile. Altering their beliefs, names, associations, speech, or physical appearance as much as possible, they adopt a life which requires that they spurn their ethnic identity—which becomes more inescapable as they try to deny it. Such persons live in fear of discovery, and although they may escape the prejudice of the majority they can never escape their inner prejudice—or the self-contempt it veils.

The most economically and cultural deprived members of the group may experience such prolonged deprivation that, like the person who suffers from chronic malnutrition, they come in time to be apathetic. Afraid to vent their wrath on the powerful majority, unable to construct a viable self-image, they turn their anger back on themselves and sink into chronic, apathetic depression. (As Huddie Ledbetter, better known as Leadbelly, once put it, "Blues got you.")

Regardless of the specific pattern, the member of a suppressed minority who projects his own hostility and self-contempt becomes hopelessly snared in neurosis. He erects internal obstacles to the satisfaction of his needs which are far more restricting than the external ones. He creates barriers where there may be none, finds rejection where he could have found acceptance, and generally limits his own freedom of choice and action. The consequences of his misdirection—added to the objective difficulties he encounters—constitute a crushing burden.

But if he understands himself and what he is seeking, even the victim of persecution can circumvent formidable barriers. He can learn to view discrimination with the kind of objectivity with which he views an accident or a business reversal: that is, as an adverse situation which can be countered best if he does not become emotionally embroiled.

Admittedly, this requires great self-knowledge and control, especially for people who have been denied the most basic opportunity for self-acceptance. The incredible thing is the number of Negroes who *have* achieved such self-understanding. Having resolved the intrapersonal problem of ethnic identity, they are free to see other facets of themselves: their occupational, professional, and community identities, their creative capacities. As they come to see themselves in broader categories, others see them more as people, less as stereotypical Negroes. These are the Negroes who make the initial break in barriers through which others are able to follow. Seeking fulfillment, not vengeance, they focus their attention on opening doors rather than on kicking at closed ones.

The Negro who has thus approached autonomy has necessarily learned to acknowledge his own residual prejudice against his people and himself. Having confronted it, he finds it a minor counterpoise to his identification with the Negro community and he can accept himself as a Negro—not as the Negro of the old stereotype, but the Negro of the new image that is emerging from the calm dignity of students sitting-in at lunch counters, from the courage of schoolchildren going to jail, from the unflinching Negroes who face attacking police dogs.

The Stinging Rebuke

It is possible for a person who has none of the objective problems of the American Negro to believe, nonetheless, that the world is totally hostile to him. There are people who live in a cloud of alienated anger and who see everyone else as inexplicably antagonistic. Their self-doubts are so encompassing that they refuse to recognize them as their own, assuming (erroneously) that acknowledging the internal source would be tantamount to accepting the validity of the judgment.

Some self-criticism is reasonable, some is not. A person may be intelligent, attractive, and potentially personable, yet feel that compared to others he is inadequate. He may discredit his capacities in the belief that the things he is are of no real significance, while the things he is not—or fears to try—are all that matter. Because his sweeping self-criticisms are patently unfair, however, he may assume that he would not make them of himself. It seems more plausible to project them onto the people around him and to interpret his unreasonable self-criticism as an unwarranted attack by others.

Continuously aware that *someone* is discrediting him and unwilling to admit who it is, he reads insult into the most innocent remark. He may respond to his projected self-contempt by unleashing an acid tongue or, fearing the consequences of aggression, he may turn his anger back on himself as chronic anxiety and depression. In either case, he feels unjustly persecuted—without being aware that the pain he feels is self-flagellation.

The adjusted American does not usually inflict this much condemnation on himself, but he is, nonetheless, prone to placing self-criticism in the mouths of others. When he does, the stage is set for tears or angry words if someone echoes his self-doubts. He is particularly likely to feel hurt when those dear to him seem to be criticizing him unfairly.

Imagine an adjusted American housewife, who has spent a rainy Saturday with the children at home, errands to run, cleaning to do, and a sense of being left out when her husband phones to say that a business engagement will detain him until after dinner. At 10:30 the children are in bed and peaceful at last, and she is cleaning the sink. At this point her husband comes home and greets her with "Haven't you finished washing the dishes *yet!*" She bursts into tears.

Her tearful response is normal, but that does not mean it is inevitable. Another wife (or the same wife on another day) might have taken the remark in stride, guessed that the business deal had probably fallen through, and mixed him a drink. Why does the first wife feel hurt?

This woman has had a trying day: that is to say, a day in which she has failed to satisfy needs. She feels an inevitable ambivalence about housework and her children, and this day her attention has been on resenting them rather than on enjoying herself in a role that she values. She feels abused. As her work drags on, she begins to suspect that it is because she is dragging her heels. She could dismiss her self-criticism and enjoy the luxury of dawdling. Or she could act on her self-criticism and enjoy dispatching her work efficiently. She does neither. Instead, she begins to imagine what her husband would say if he arrived home before her work is done.

She has been tense all day (for she has been failing to meet her needs), and now this tension takes form as hurt indignation about the unfair criticism her husband would voice—if he were there to voice it. (A simple rule of thumb is that whatever criticism one imagines someone else may be thinking, or would think if he knew about something, is projected self-criticism.)

Her projection becomes prophecy. She is still at the sink when her husband comes in and speaks the lines she has prepared for him. Her *intra*personal conflict teeters on the edge of *inter*personal quarrel. Wanting to avert the quarrel (and perhaps to shame her husband) she turns her anger into tears. Another wife might have thrown the coffeepot at his head, in an equally disfunctional response to projected self-criticism.

It should be noted that not all unjust accusations sting. Those criticisms which the individual does not apply to himself will strike him as surprising, incredible, or amusing. He can mull on such a charge, see if there is any basis for it, then either act on it or dismiss is without rancor. *The unfair criticism which galls is that which he directs against himself.* Projected onto others it becomes the basis of hurt feelings, especially if someone emotionally significant to him invites the projection by voicing a similar criticism.

The Martyr

There is no inherent misdirection in holding unorthodox views. Indeed, the autonomous individual, free from compulsive conformance and unquestioned assumptions, is likely to be unorthodox. And in an era characterized by a progressive disintegration of the *status quo* and a frightening paucity of constructive alternatives, there is a desperate need for creative, unorthodox thinkers. They stimulate the climate of controversy without which political democracy becomes an empty formalism.

Yet tragically, the advocacy of unorthodox ideas in contemporary America is more often a symptom of neurosis than the result of autonomous thought. The radicalism which misdirection engenders is more likely to lead to sterile rebellion than to constructive leadership. The resultant loss is both individual and social, and the misdirections and neuroses of the unorthodox assume the stature of a major social problem.

One of the most common irrational motivations to

unorthodox behavior is rebellion against parental and social authority. Rebellion is a means by which the individual (especially the adolescent and young adult) explores, establishes, and experiences his individuality. As such it is functional, especially in an urban-industrial society where a high degree of individuation is required for a full and meaningful life.

But the rebel who fails to understand the motives and function of his rebellion is likely to confuse the issue. He will in all probability fail to exploit the opportunities for growth which rebellion offers and become preoccupied with rebellion for its own sake. When rebellion becomes an end in itself, it offers few rewards to the individual and gives a purely negative cast to his thought and action. He is no longer seeking new solutions, but only hacking at the old answers.

Rebellion usually bogs down in neurotic misdirection when it involves a self-imposed martyrdom. A case in point is the young radical who espouses unpopular ideas with the expectation that he will be persecuted. Finding everyone around him tinged with the hostility he projects, he retaliates by flinging back ideas which he has learned make most people uncomfortable. He expresses unpopular ideas because he believes in them, but he believes in them partly because they are unpopular.

Expecting to be met with hostility, he enters any situation fully prepared to counterattack. His antagonistic approach continuously invites other people to project their own hostility onto him and to respond to it with annoyance and indignation. Moreover, most people he meets have at least some sympathy with his views (the ambivalent echo of their own orthodoxy) but are uneasy at finding heretical thoughts in the corners of their conventional minds. They are only too glad to project their radical potential onto this unpleasant young man and to despise him for it. As he loudly proclaims himself the spokesman for his cause, the hostility which his aggressive behavior invites reflects on this cause, and he harms that which he purports to defend.

Such advocates of the unorthodox are likely to be individuals who fear that they are inherently unlikable. For such a person, taking an unpopular stand can be a means of deliberately giving others a specific reason to dislike him. Assuming that others would be hostile to him in any case, he seems to find some consolation in believing that he is disliked for his ideas— which he could change if he wished. As long as he never puts it to the test, he can hope that recanting would make him acceptable. Meanwhile he can savor his image as a lonely martyr—which he finds much more to his liking than the image of himself as the fellow nobody likes.

A sure symptom of this neurosis is the effort such individuals make to be certain that other people know about their unorthodox views as soon as possible on making their acquaintance. They are prone to whipping out their opinions, apropos of nothing at all, merely to flaunt them publicly. Because they value the unpopularity of their ideas, they are unlikely to do much to further general acceptance of these views, regardless of their protestations. They are more interested in shocking than in communicating.

Just as the conformist harbors latent radical sympathies, so the misdirected martyr has a residual conventionality. In his protracted assault on the *status quo*, he takes increasingly extreme and uncompromising stands. But the more extreme his position, the more outraged is the conventional side of his ambivalence, and the harder he will find it to accept himself.

Meanwhile, not only is his need for self-acceptance blocked, but his need for association also becomes difficult to satisfy. Pursuing his ideological attack, he is unlikely to find meaningful association with people of more conventional persuasion and his interaction with other radicals is likely to center on mighty controversies over minuscule differences of opinion. As his deprivation mounts, his tension also rises and his fanaticism flames.

As gadflies on the body politic, such people may serve a function. However misguided and maladroit, they at least keep controversy alive. It is the autonomous individual who is desperately needed, however. The person who has a basic acceptance of himself and a developed capacity for enjoying the things he does and the people he is among can explain the rational considerations which have led him to his position in an atmosphere that encourages others to consider his views. And he is free to sort ideas on their merits, not limited to choosing among them as weapons.

But Words Can Never Hurt Me

Projection does not rid the individual of self-contempt and hostility. On the contrary it leads him to feel surrounded by contemptuous, hostile people. Refusing to accept the inner source of self-contempt, he responds to it in ways which are inevitably misdirected. He may try to mitigate it by ingratiating himself with others: he may retaliate, he may weep because he dares not retaliate, or he my cry *mea culpa*. In any case, he does nothing to improve his own poor opinion of himself.

The adjusted American fears incurring the disapproval of others. Yet even vilification cannot undermine a secure self-acceptance. Whatever difficulties the hostility of others may impose, it does not in itself elicit a passionate response in the individual. It is an objective phenomenon and can be dealt with accordingly. The criticism that stings is self-criticism. The hostility that engulfs and terrifies is projected by the individual himself and is simply a measure of his unfilled needs.

In discussing hatred in chapter 4, we pointed out that the criticism which A hurls at B is unconscious autobiography. Here it should be added that if B is annoyed by A's criticism, it is only because he concurs. He may in fact find a sense of relief at having such a plausible place to hang his self-contempt— if he can discredit the source, he hopes to rid himself of the doubt. Just as the prejudiced require their scapegoats, so the victims may seek out their tormentors.

6

INDIRECT
SELF-ACCEPTANCE

Whatever they undertake becomes a passionate pursuit; but they never arrive, never pause. They demonstrate the fact that we can never have enough of that which we really do not want, and that we run fastest and farthest when we run from ourselves. ERIC HOFFER

One normal neurosis seems to dominate the personality of the adjusted American. More than any other single factor, it is responsible for his insatiably accumulative, tensely gregarious life-style. Riesman coined the phrase "other-direction" and struck a responsive chord with Americans. They seized on the phrase, for it seemed to name and to delineate something basic in their fellows—and in themselves. Riesman observed that diffuse anxiety is the salient characteristic of the "other-directed." And as we have seen, anxiety is a symptom of unfilled need. *The Lonely Crowd,* however, was focused on the interaction between social change and characterological transformation. It did not attempt to explain what basic needs the anxiety-ridden, "other-directed" American was failing to satisfy, or why he failed to satisfy them. This task remains to be undertaken. *Why* are Americans so hungry for the approval of others?

The adjusted American lacks *self*-approval; that is to say, he has not developed a self-image that he can believe is both accurate and acceptable. To do so he would require successful techniques for creating an accurate and acceptable self-image through honest introspection, candid association, and meaningful activity. The patterns to which he has adjusted do not include such techniques. Instead, the culture abounds with misdirections, which the adjusted American acquires. There are the patterns of alienation and projection discussed above, through which he seeks to deny unpalatable aspects of himself. But perhaps above all he learns to seek self-acceptance indirectly, by seeking to substitute the good opinion of others for self-approval. It is thus that he becomes "other-directed."

Half certain of his own inadequacy, he attempts to present himself to others in an appealing way. When (or if) he has won their approval he hopes that they will be able to convince him that he is a better man than *he* thinks he is.

But this quest for indirect self-acceptance is fundamentally misdirected. In chapter 3 we discussed the self needs, noting that the individual needs association with other people in order that they may be his mirrors, his models, and the recipients of his actions. The striving for approval, which is the crux of the attempt to achieve indirect self-acceptance, is a distorted, ineffectual substatute for the mirror function of association.

Reflected in the responses of the people around him the individual sees an image of himself. The perspectives of himself gained from others help him to evaluate his self-image, to have confidence in his virtues, to admit the existence of his defects. This process requires openness and honesty both in the individual's self-scrutiny and in his approach to others, for *the opinion of others can contribute to self-acceptance only when the individual believes that others see him as he really is.* Otherwise, he cannot give credence to the image he sees reflected in their eyes.

But the person who is caught up in the quest for indirect self-acceptance is more concerned with making a favorable impression on others than with seeing an honest reflection of himself. He attempts to manipulate the way he appears to others. Consequently he cannot credit any favorable image they may reflect, for he has good reason to think what he sees is only his most flattering angle.

Moreover, he is likely to become preoccupied with the limitations he is struggling to conceal from others, with the result that these "defects" loom disproportionately large in his self-image. The person who seeks indirect self-acceptance thus begins by trying to manipulate the image he presents to others and ends by having a distorted self-image, in which his defects are magnified.

The adjusted American enters this hall of distorting mirrors in childhood. It is not merely that he fails to learn techniques for achieving self-acceptance; he is virtually forced to find himself unacceptable. The image of an acceptable person which the child learns in the typical middle-class American home is a fraud. It is not and can never be the image of any existing person. Rather, the image is a figment of middle-class proprieties in its general outlines and the specific self-deceptions of parents in its details.

The typical middle-class American child learns that an "acceptable" child would not do, or even *want* to do, certain things. Hurting the baby, biting his mother, playing with excrement, playing with his genitals, playing with his playmates' genitals—there are a great many things which he is taught are shameful even to think about doing. Yet inevitably he does think about doing such things and (depending on how vigilant his mother is) may do them at times. He could have learned that it is not unusual to feel like doing such things, but that in the family—and society—of which he is a member, such things are simply not the custom. Instead, he is led to believe that his "nasty" inclinations set him apart from other people as a "dirty" boy.

As he grows older he is taught to believe that a "good" child (or a "normal" one, depending on family usage) would not resent his parents considering all they have done for him and how much *they* love *him*. Yet the dynamics of childhood are such that any child must inevitably feel a certain amount of resentment toward his parents. (This is a complicated pattern that will be discussed at length in chapter 11.) Thus a vicious syllogism is established: only evil children ever hate their parents; sometimes I hate my parents; therefore I am an evil child.

Once in school, the middle-class American child is pressured to achieve, both scholastically and socially. If his performance is less than outstanding (if he is not in the advanced reading group, or does not qualify for the enrichment program), he will soon be aware that he is a disappointment to his parents. If he has not corrected his deficiencies by high school (that is, if he is not an honor student, a star halfback, and very popular), he is led to believe that he has bungled his opportunities, that he is already a failure.

In short, the child is presented with a phony image of an "acceptable child," less as a model than as a point of invidious comparison. No one ever seriously thought he could measure up to it, yet somehow he is condemned because he does not. Moreover, the adult roles that he is led to idealize are sham. From the mass media he draws his heroes: the little child tries to imitate the heroes of the TV Western, the adolescent emulates the virile men (or the glamorous girls) of the cigarette commercials. But these images are unrelated to the lives and experiences of real people. Taking these as his models, it is not surprising that the child finds himself unable to measure up to these phony images of what is manly or (womanly).

By the time the child arrives at puberty, quickening sexual interests lead him to further self-contempt. The feeling of being "dirty" induced by parental horror at his childhood sex play comes surging forward. His parents are unlikely to be comfortable with their own sexuality and are consequently quick to add to, rather than to alleviate, the child's sense of shame.

Throughout this "happy" childhood, the anxiety-ridden youth is discovering himself, and discovering that he is in large measure unacceptable. Faltering, he clutches at what seems to be support. As his parents plant the seeds of his self-doubts, they nonetheless insist that they love him. The child clings to this straw, and attempts to substitute the affection of his parents for his missing self-acceptance.

His parents are most likely to proffer their love when he successfully conceals certain facets of himself (above all, feelings and desires which the parents have never learned to accept in themselves). Thus the child learns to seek indirect self-acceptance, to present a less than candid picture of himself to others in the hope of winning their approval and thereby easing his self-doubts.

In some cases, a child is convinced that his parents have an unalterably low opinion of him. Such a child may practice as much parent-avoidance as possible and concentrate on seeking approval from other adults (teachers, coaches, etc.) or from a peer group. Winning the admiration of his gang may thus also become a misdirected substitute for seeking self-acceptance directly.

By the time a youth has been transformed into an adult, his thirst for approval seems insatiable. But to borrow a phrase from Hoffer, he can never have enough of that which he really does not need. He needs *self*-acceptance, and however much of his talent, energy, and possessions are committed to the struggle to win approval from others, self-acceptance cannot be achieved thereby. There is a fundamental defect in the method.

Anxious Conformity

The attempt to achieve indirect self-acceptance may take the form of conformity, through which an individual seeks approval and acceptance by others. Some conformity merely reflects the fact that the individual has acquired the customs of his particular region, class, or ethnic group. This is simple conventionality, and although it limits the individual's perception of alternatives and narrows his self-image it is not usually motivated by the quest for indirect self-acceptance. When conformity *is* motivated by this quest, it has an undercurrent of anxiety.

The person who is simply conventional has some difficulty in imagining himself being very different from those around him. In contrast, the conscious conformist sees himself as significantly different from those whose acceptance he craves. He tries to conceal these differences in his attempt to fit into the group and to emulate (or simulate) those characteristics that he believes the group finds acceptable.

The conscious conformist uses a great deal of ingenuity in ascertaining the behaviors, opinions, and characteristics of a member in good standing of the groups where he seeks acceptance. He then molds his own behaviors, opinions, and characteristics accordingly. The cut of his suit, the brand of his necktie, the novels he reads, the causes he is identified with are all determined by careful observation of trends among the people he wants to accept him. He wants to be "in."

He may go well beyond the externals of dress and manner and become highly sensitized to the expectations and responses of others. This enables him to adapt his behavior to subtle and shifting patterns, but always with a watchful eye on the impression his actions make on others, always carefully withholding a great deal of himself.

Not all who seek to achieve upward mobility by conformity to the expectations of a higher class level have such skills. However, if they have enough money, they can hire people who do have the skills to teach them the formulas. There is even a department store (in Texas, of course) where people who have suddenly acquired wealth but have not yet attuned themselves to the most prestigious ways of spending it can hire taste. For a stiff fee, experts will choose for them a wardrobe, a house (in a selected neighborhood), furnishings and décor, and arrange for speech lessons to complete the transformation—*Pygmalion* come to life!

Such conscious conformists differ from the usual social climber in method if not motive: the old-fashioned climber typically seeks to attach himself to persons of high status and prestige; the conscious conformist seeks to fit himself to a pattern of tastes and behaviors which he believes characterizes persons of high status and prestige. He is chagrined by those tastes and habits which he discovers in himself that bear the lingering imprint of his lower-middle-class (or working-class) origins. He believes that these traces of an earlier self are inappropriate to his present level of affluence and sophistication, and he conceals—perhaps from everyone but himself—the residual characteristics he finds embarrassing. (A case in point is a fellow who has cultivated a polished Harvard inflection but has to be careful at cocktail parties because after the fifth highball he lapses into a Southern Appalachian twang.)

The vestiges of what the conscious conformist once was could coexist peacefully with what he has become, but he believes that they invalidate the image he has so carefully cultivated. He builds a public image that he can never permit to be casual or revealing. And herein lies the futility of seeking self-acceptance in this indirect fashion: whatever acceptance the conformist may be granted by others, he attributes to his façade. He remains uncomfortable with the self he has hidden behind it. Small wonder that under the surface of his apparently suave life style there runs a chronic anxiety.

Popularity

The person who achieves widespread acceptance—the popular individual—has won what others covet, and the others believe that he must be content. Some popular people are, but these are the exceptional few who are popular because they are accepting of themselves —and hence of others. It is their ability to make other people feel accepted and comfortable that draws people to them. *Such people are popular because they are self-accepting and not the other way around.*

The person who tries to reverse the causal sequence and seeks popularity as an indirect means to self-acceptance is likely to achieve neither. And even if he does become popular, proceeding in the same general manner as his compatriots but having the good luck and adroitness to win widespread admiration, he is caught in a misdirection. If it were possible for the quest for indirect self-acceptance to be rewarding, this person should be fulfilled. But his hard-won popularity does not eliminate his self-doubts.

Seeking indirect self-acceptance through popularity, he has tried to disguise, rather than to alter, what he believes are his defects. He presents to others a mask, a retouched likeness of himself which minimizes some features and exaggerates others. He attributes his popularity to his skill as a masker and thus precludes from the outset finding in popularity proof of acceptability. What his public admires, he fears is counterfeit.

And there are always some who are not counted among his admirers, some who are quick to point out his faults, to peer through the cracks in his mask. Over the applause of his public, the popular person often hears clearly those carping detractors who echo his self-doubts. Moreover, the popularity he has won may prove a liability by leading him to cling to the palliative it offers, rather than to abandon the indirect approach and seek self-acceptance directly. Having achieved what he thought was his goal, he is busy refurbishing the techniques by which he arrived, hopeful that someday they will bring him fulfillment.

Success

Man can find direct self-acceptance through the actions by which he tests his capacities, verifies and expands his self-image, and experiences desired aspects of himself. But when he acts primarily to impress others, he becomes involved once again in the futile quest for indirect self-acceptance. He becomes preoccupied with the recognition that others may accord him, hoping that their recognition will enable him to think better of himself.

The person who seeks indirect self-acceptance through recognition is likely to concentrate his energies where he is most confident of succeeding. This would be logical if success were sufficient to satisfy his need. It is not. His need is to verify and expand an acceptable self-image, and the pursuit of success rapidly becomes a misdirection. As he pursues success he is likely to become increasingly proficient in areas where he has little doubt of his capacity and to relegate to the limbo of untried potential many capacities he would like to experience in himself.

Self-acceptance comes only to those who have the courage to investigate the areas where their self-doubts reside. Viewed a little differently, many self-doubts represent uncertainty about one's ability to do something one regards as important. The person who seeks self-acceptance *directly* is motivated to try such things, to explore his potential and develop his capacities.

But the adjusted American pursuing success is least likely to venture in those areas where he has the greatest self-doubt. Fearing to appear ludicrous or inept he avoids those activities in which he is uncertain of himself. Because these are precisely the areas in which he longs to excel, the races he fears to enter seem to him more significant than the ones he wins. (A man may earn a doctorate, for example, but doubt his capacity for intimate association. In all likelihood he will respond to his fears by burying himself in further research.)

The man who competes only in those activities where he feels most confident of success finds failure acutely painful. If he fails in the area where he feels most competent, he is left with a sense of total inadequacy. It is because he has so much at stake that failure leads him to react with disproportionate anger or depression. And if he survives the initial contest, he must face ever stiffer competition and suffer increasing anxiety about failure. He finds that people forget quickly and that he must achieve ever more difficult feats, must pursue ever-receding objectives. So long as he seeks to substitute success for self-acceptance he must keep on succeeding.

Those who do not fail but yet do not achieve the height of their ambitions (and ambition necessarily outruns achievement) find themselves in an ambiguous situation. They may not be certain that they have failed, but they know that they have not succeeded as they had hoped. The myth is that success is open to all Americans, yet inevitably most are left with a sense of disappointment and a haunting fear of inadequacy.

The quest for recognition may lead to the pursuit of a specific award (a promotion, a championship) or of privileges and perquisites (a private office, an unlimited expense account). The attempt to impress others with what one can do thus often becomes an attempt to impress others with the symbols of prowess. The trophies of achievement or the spoils of successful business ventures are symbols displayed to others to show the worth of the individual who was able to seize them—as Veblen long since observed.

In certain African tribes a man who kills a lion can put an iron pot on his roof to symbolize the kill, and the worth of the hunter is counted in pots. In Western culture, too, the skill of the successful predator is displayed symbolically—not by pots on the roof perhaps, but by other items of value and above all by money. It is not, however, the possession of wealth as such that impresses, but rather the power of wealth to command goods and services. (The wealthy miser living in squalor is not accorded esteem.) The person who tries to impress others with his ability to command goods and services consumes conspicuously and wastefully. The canons of taste change, and conspicuous display is less blatant in America of the 1960's than it was at the turn of the century. But conspicuous waste has become the cornerstone of the American economy (enforced obsolescence through model change is only one example). Veblen's analyses are fundamentally as appropriate to modern Americans as to the captains of industry of the last century.

When goods are consumed not for satisfaction but primarily for the impression consumption makes on others, it is not surprising if the consumer is insatiable. Nor is it surprising if he seeks to inflate his worth in the eyes of others by consuming beyond his means. But that such consumption leads to more anxiety than pleasure is a frequently observed fact.

The quest for success or for the appearance of affluence is thus another variant of the quest for indirect self-acceptance. It is behavior which cannot satisfy the need that motivates it—a classic example of misdirection.

The Pervasive Neurosis

The struggle to achieve indirect self-acceptance is a pervasive pattern of American normalcy—a very normal neurosis. Not all seek indirect self-acceptance in the same way, but wherever they are and whatever they are doing, adjusted Americans devote the major share of their time, energy, and assets to seeking the acceptance and approval of others. They may debate the best means of making a favorable impression, but they never seem to doubt that this is an important goal.

Yet the quest for indirect self-acceptance is inevitably bound up with a sense that one's "real" self is unacceptable. Attempts to gloss over defects of which the individual is painfully aware or to feign capacities which he doubts are real only make it more difficult for him to accept himself.

Paradoxically, often pathetically, other people may recognize and tolerate characteristics which an individual has been trying to conceal. For example, a man trying to hide the fact that he lacks formal education may never realize that his friends are aware he is largely self-educated, admire him for it, and make allowances for the gaps in his intellectual background. But in spite of such acceptance by others, so long as the individual is afraid of being himself he cannot believe that he is acceptable.

There are even instances in which characteristics a person believes he is only feigning have become real, without his quite becoming aware of that fact. For instance, the effective intellectual fraud is forced to read and think in order to maintain the illusion. He may ultimately become an intellectual without being aware of his metamorphosis. So long as he thinks that what he does is only sham, a pretense kept up in order to impress others, he cannot credit his own growth.

Thus the quest for indirect self-acceptance leads away from self-knowledge and often increases the sense of inadequacy which the individual is trying to overcome. The person who distorts the image he presents to others discredits in advance any approval which may be bestowed on him. To the extent that he succeeds in manipulating the opinion others have of him, he convinces himself that they perceive him inaccurately—and thus he sabotages one of the basic means of verifying an acceptable self-image.

Inevitably, the pursuit of indirect self-acceptance produces an exaggerated concern with outward appearance. It leads a man to feign a friendliness he does not feel, rather than to develop his capacity for warmth. It leads a woman to feel that her grooming, but not her self, is acceptable. It leads to anxious conformity and to a tense struggle for recognition. It lies behind the spending on overextended credit through which Americans try to achieve an impressive life style. It leads to the fake, to a mode of existence that, like a Hollywood set, is only an elaborate front with nothing behind but a few props to shore it up.

Meanwhile, the really basic need for self-acceptance remains unfulfilled. Assuming that his need is for acceptance by others, the American does not learn how to accept himself.

7
SOLITARY CONFINEMENT

*He could have resigned himself to a prison. To end as
a prisoner—that could be a life's ambition. But it was
a barred cage that he was in. Calmly and insolently, as
if at home, the din of the world streamed out and in
through the bars, the prisoner was really free, he could
take part in everything, nothing that went on outside
escaped him, he could simply have left the cage, the
bars were yards apart, he was not even a prisoner.*

FRANZ KAFKA

A man can be safely subjected to solitary confinement
for limited intervals only. Long periods in solitary
tend to induce personality disintegration or outright
madness, since the fulfillment of the basic need for
association is effectively blocked. The adjusted American lives almost constantly within sight or earshot of
others but nevertheless spends much of his time in a
psychological solitary confinement. Some people even
contrive to serve life sentences—with results that
might be anticipated. The paradox of the "lonely
crowd" exists because Americans render most of their
associations strained, superficial, and unsatisfying.
Their confinement, like that of Kafka's prisoner, is
self-imposed.

When confronted with an adverse environment,
some microrganisms seal themselves off to await bet-

ter times. In an analogous fashion, many people assume that their social environment is adverse and encyst themselves psychologically. Fearing that open and candid association might be damaging, they erect barriers against it. Their walls are well constructed and difficult to breach. But the dangers are illusory, and the walls serve to confine rather than to protect.

Behind These Walls

The individual may refuse to admit the defensive nature of the barriers he places between himself and others. He may attribute his loneliness to external circumstance; one such rationalization is the pressure of a job. Here is the man immersed in his profession, who says he would like close friends but has no time to cultivate them. It may be, as he claims, that by driving himself he has risen rapidly. But so have others who devote less of their total lives to their work and delegate much that this man does by himself. It is not that his career demands so much of him, but rather that he demands so much of his career.

He makes certain that he has no free time in order to insulate himself from unstructured association with others. In his business contacts he displays the surface warmth that his professional role requires, but he carefully confines the interaction to that stylized relationship. If inveigled into a social situation, he still contrives to play his professional role, for he fears casual intimacy. (Here is the professor who approaches a cockatil party as if it were a seminar and debates esoteric matters with anyone willing to play the game. And here, too, is the doctor who maintains his clinical attitude in the most casual social gathering.) Behind the mask of the profession, self-doubts proliferate.

Yet such a man needs to explore his self-potential through candid association even more than the next person. Because he deprives himself of intimate association he experiences chronic tension, the physiological response to deprivation. He misdirects this drive, channeling it back into his career. The more deprived he is the harder he works, but not toward the satisfaction of his need.

Flight from association into work is only one of many devices by which people seek to avoid intimacy. Their motive is fear—fear of the possible consequences of revealing too much about themselves. But their concern is largely unwarranted. It is true that in some instances an individual might expose himself to palpable harm by revealing certain aspects of himself. The criminal, the sexual deviant, or the political heretic, for example, finds it advisable to withhold certain aspects of himself in most associations. The typical American, however, has few dark secrets which he must guard at his peril. Most of *his* supposed aberrations are facets of the self which are common, perhaps even universal. Other people are struggling to disguise precisely the same thoughts or potentialities.

The typical American shrinks from candid intimacy less from fear of prosecution than from fear of rejection. It is true that people who are themselves concealing certain potential may be agitated when someone else flaunts similar behaviors and desires. But how the self is presented—defiantly or with warmth, defensively or with self-acceptance—is the critical factor in determining how it will be received. In a situation where they do not feel threatened themselves, most people can be accepting of most aspects of other people.

In any event, association can be open and candid on the whole even though some aspects of the self are not brought forward. It is less a question of how much of the self is revealed than a question of motive. It is one thing to withhold facets of the self for fear of rejection and quite another to withhold facets of the self because they are likely to impede the enjoyment of a particular association. The individual may have capacities which are not germane to a particular interaction; indeed, the multifaceted individual could not possibly experience his total self in any given situation. But this does not have to interfere with his enjoyment of others. For example, the adult enjoys interacting with children, even though he does not call to the fore many facets of himself which he finds inappropriate to the relationship. The critical point is that he is not uncomfortable about the facets of himself which he withholds in interacting with the child.

People who are self-accepting have no anxiety about the aspects of themselves which are not apparent at a given moment. They are not worried about what might slip out unbidden. They bring forth largely those elements of the self that are likely to facilitate their enjoyment of a particular situation not because they are hiding other potential, but rather because they are seeking to derive the greatest amount of pleasure from their present company. As a result, they find rewards in even the most limited association. They are comfortable with other people because they are first of all comfortable with themselves.

In contrast, the person who is uncomfortable or bored with most other people is uncomfortable with a great many facets of himself. He is uneasy about the potential he withholds from others, and he erects defensive barriers to hold them at a distance. Usually he manages to rationalize these barriers: he is too busy to find time for friends, or the people around him come from a different background and have nothing in common with him, or the people around him are unfriendly and have shut him out. Whatever the rationalization, the reason he maintains his defenses is fear of what candid intimacy might reveal about himself.

Retreat from Insight

Often the individual erects walls less to conceal things from others than to block insight. This pattern is exemplified by a student who lives in the riotous intimacy of a fraternity house, yet manages to be lonely. He has convinced himself that the companionship he requires is *intellectual* companionship, and he finds his fraternity brothers interested largely in sports, women, and beer. Outside the fraternity he finds much the same situation (being the same young man). The girls he knows are as shallow as his fraternity brothers; worse yet, the self-styled intellectuals he encounters seem transparent frauds. In short, he finds no one who seems a suitable companion, and he remains aloof, waiting for the "rare spirit" who could offer him companionship.

His self-imposed isolation is a defensive measure. He is attempting to become an intellectual by denying other facets of himself, thus restricting rather than broadening his self-image. He has alienated his capacity to enjoy such things as fraternity picnics, football games, and bull sessions. The shallowness he deplores in his fraternity brothers is his own projection; whether or not the projection fits, what this student perceives is his own rejected interests.

He senses that intimate association with the fraternity brothers he scorns might make it apparent that he is not so different from them as he would like to be. Out of fear of what he might discover about himself in association with them, he closes the door. His desire for an idealized intellectual companion serves to rationalize remaining at a safe distance from revealing association, but it leaves him bored and lonely. And never having learned how to interact comfortably, he would probably plunge into awkward silence or equally awkward monologue if he ever did encounter such a "rare spirit."

Thus some people isolate themselves in order to avert the insight that intimate association facilitates. The recluse, however, is less common among Americans than another type: the person who is afraid of candid intimacy, but is terrified of solitude.

The person who is afraid to inquire too closely into his own motives and desires often finds a host of unbidden thoughts crowding into his mind when he is alone. The inner rage he fears to acknowledge, the alienated sadistic desires he shrinks from, seem to take form as a Thing that lurks in an empty room, that stirs in the far from silent house, that spies him out from the darkness beyond the window. So he (more likely she) draws the blinds, turns up the volume on the television set so that people's voices fill the room, or seizes the telephone and calls a friend. Anything to escape the potentialities of solitude.

Many people who are less inclined to tremble at shadows are nonetheless afraid of insight and try to avoid it by surrounding themselves with people. Trying to evade both candid association and introspective solitude, they envelop themselves in a pseudo-intimacy. Such a person maintains walls as impregnable as those put up by the recluse, but camouflages them with a spurious gregariousness. Like a whirling dervish he seeks escape from the self—but his whirl is social.

He may seek the superficial intimacy generated by the habitués of the country club lounge. This is a withholding kind of togetherness, which screens each participant behind a stylized interaction. There is an air of *entre nous* in these gatherings; speech is rapid and continuous as if people feared leaving an empty space into which insight might slip. The conversation, like a cunningly contrived gown, seems to reveal precisely that which it safely conceals.

For another social class the setting may be the morning coffee session or the evening at a neighborhood tavern, but the dilaogue serves the same function. It consists of safely innocuous small talk: stock opinions on world events, sports, weather, public figures, recent scandals, television—or quotations from other equally vapid conversations. It conveys the impression of intimacy without ever baring the self.

Association such as this serves only as a diversion. If it is not available, the nearest book, magazine, or crossword puzzle can be substituted. Association that is largely interchangeable with entertainment cannot fulfill the individual; it can only insulate him equally from the self-discovery possible in candid association and from the self-scrutiny possible in solitude. When used as a means of numbing self-awareness, association becomes merely an anesthetic.

The Wrong Door

Some people sentence themselves to solitary confinement because they confuse the need for association with another need. A common example is the confusion of the need for association with the need for food. Companionship and food are associated in the individual's mind by years of simultaneous satisfaction; in infancy being fed and being cuddled occur together, and throughout life the dinner table is a focal point of intimacy. People expect more than physical sustenance from a meal, an expectation which underlies the common dislike for eating alone. But the person who is generally deprived of association may make eating a symbol for the intimacy he craves.

The prodigiously fat girl is likely to be involved in this misdirection and its concomitant problems. Although she may have many appealing qualities, her fat complicates her social relations. Only an occasional boy dates her (although others might like to if they did not fear the jibes of their friends) and those who do ask her out are often boys who obviously have few other opportunities. Typically, she is not content with the leavings and prefers not to date at all. Girls may be less concerned about her appearance, but since social activities usually involve couples she is often left out by them as well.

Aware that she is lonely, she nevertheless fails to connect her loneliness with the tense craving she feels. She makes a mental leap from companionship to food. Instead of heading for the front door in search of friends, she waddles to the refrigerator door in search of a snack.

Like most misdirected actions, her behavior involves a vicious circle. The more acute her loneliness, the more she tries to allay her craving by stuffing herself. The more she eats, the fatter she grows and the more her weight interferes with her relations with others. And then the more her fat impairs her association, the more acute her need becomes, and the more she eats. Thus her misdirection almost literally feeds itself.

There is another neurotic motive in her pattern. Tension is customarily interpreted as anger by Americans, and this girl is no exception. She translates her needfulness into anger as well as hunger. But fearing that overt hostility would make a bad situation worse, she plays the jolly fat girl whenever she is around people and turns her desire to hurt others into self-destructiveness. Eating is the form of self-destruction that she understands best.

Keep Your Damn Jack

Another common barrier to meaningful association is bristling independence, manifested in a refusal to accept any favor that cannot be returned immediately or to incur a debt that cannot readily be canceled. Here is the man who insists on picking up the check 51 percent of the time, but despises people who allow him to pay it 52 percent of the time. He voices intense aversion to anyone who exploits a friend. Indignation betrays the projection of an alienated desire—in this instance, a desire to be dependent.

This man is likely to equate being dependent on people with being accepted by them. Such equations originate in childhood when parents stress that they do things for their child because they love him and withhold favors to show disapproval. The child comes to believe that the things others do for him are the proof of his acceptability to them, and he may cling to this conviction throughout his life. Thus the desire to be dependent is rooted in hope for indirect self-acceptance. (The reasoning runs as follows: "If people accepted me, maybe I could accept myself. If people accepted me, they would show it by doing nice things for me. Therefore, if people would do nice things for me, maybe I could accept myself.")

Typically, however, the adult learns to regard dependence as a symptom of immaturity and alienates his desire to be dependent. Moreover, if he comes to doubt that others could like him enough to do things for him, the stage is set for compulsive independence. He abandons the quest for indirect self-acceptance through dependency (often to seek indirect self-acceptance through recognition) for he fears the humiliation of asking and not receiving. Yet his desire to be dependent persists, for this neurotic pattern was learned in childhood, and it has been alienated, not lost. In an attempt to rid himself of his desire to be dependent, he projects it onto anyone who invites it —perhaps he had a demanding wife or a parasitic brother-in-law.

The person who alienates and projects a desire to be dependent would not, in all probability, find the behavior rewarding if he tried it. He needs self-acceptance and candid association, and having others peel his grapes would not satisfy these needs. He has little opportunity to discover this, however, for he is busy keeping the record of favors straight and balanced. He cannot enter into an easy give-and-take and may even find it impossible to accept help when he really needs it. What he thinks is pride is only reluctance to accept a favor.

There is a story about a man who had a flat tire on a lonely road and discovered that his jack was missing. Seeing a farmhouse on the hill, he set out to borrow a jack. But the idea of asking a stranger for help bothered him, and shortly he began to wonder if the farmer would be willing to lend him a jack. The more he thought about it the less likely it seemed. Yet this seemed a shabby way to treat a man in trouble—after all, he was not going to steal the jack. By the time he reached the farmyard his embarrassment had become indignation. When the farmer opened to his knock, the man snapped, "I just came to tell you that you can keep your damn jack!"

Preaching the Wall

Whatever mechanism he employs, the lonely American is isolated behind walls of his own construction. Yet the same withdrawn individual is often strangely gregarious in circumstances of physical discomfort or danger. The passengers on a snowbound train may feel a twinge of regret when the tracks are cleared. In their daily lives, Americans are preoccupied with the quest for indirect self-acceptance—pursuing success or higher class status or popularity or just the neighbors' good opinion—and fail to associate candidly lest they jeopardize the illusions they are trying to maintain. A crisis diverts their attention from their usual concern with concealing much of themselves, and provides an excuse for interacting with strangers. Particularly if they assume that they will never again encounter their companions in crisis, they may suspend efforts to make a favorable impression. Under these circumstances they venture out from behind their walls and they are amply rewarded. But they almost invariably fail to perceive why, and retreat from candid association again as soon as they resume their daily routine.

The camaraderie of combat infantrymen is a classic instance of intimate association in crisis. The warm relationship common among men under fire is rare in civilian life. Yet the comrades-in-arms who are recalled with nostalgia were a random collection, brought together with no regard for the criteria by which intimate associates are usually chosen. Clearly, it is not the personalities involved which explain the bond.

During combat, men are more concerned with staying alive than with the impression they are making. For that matter, the total lack of privacy in life at close quarters makes it essentially impossible to maintain illusions. Moreover, those men who successfully adapt to combat have proved to themselves that they can do what must be done despite fear; they have verified the aspects of their self-image which are most crucial in their immediate situation. Far more than in most friendships, men who are together under fire feel that they know and accept themselves and their companions. Of necessity trusting each other with their lives, they manage also to trust each other with an honest view of themselves.

There is something absurd about holding back from association until the fear of death eclipses the fear of people. The person who recognizes how little he has to fear from intimate association and how much he needs it readily escapes from the solitary confinement to which others unwittingly sentence themselves. As a character in an O'Neill play observes, "Man's loneliness is but his fear of life." [1]

8

SEXUALIZATION

Intense sexual desire, too, can be caused not by physiological but by psychic needs. An insecure person who has an intense need to prove his worth to himself, to show others how irresistible he is, or to dominate others by "making" them sexually, will easily feel intense sexual desires . . . [and] will be prone to think that the intensity of his desires is due to the demands of his body, while actually these are determined by his psychic needs. ERICH FROMM

Like most cultures with ascetic roots, American culture has a strong sexual undercurrent. One consequence is that sexual interpretations have become conventional explanations for anything an individual does not understand or does not choose to face. Freud pointed to the way in which sexual desires masqueraded as other needs in the Victorian era, but little attention has been devoted to the way in which other needs masquerade as sexual desire in the Freudian era. *The tendency to regard as sexual desire needs which are actually nonsexual in nature we shall term sexualization.* The ensuing behaviors may lead to sexual gratification, but are not likely to fulfill the other needs motivating the individual. Needs which are sexualized are usually deprived.

The Wolf

There is a type of human male that has been known in various cultures at various times as a rake, a roué, a libertine, but Americans usually refer to him by the common name of "wolf." The Wolf spends most of his leisure in pursuit of female companions for his bed. His affairs are brief, and he boasts that his aim is the seduction of as many girls as possible, while avoiding all serious entanglements. Because of his reputation as a seducer it is often assumed that he has a more intense sexual drive than more conventional men.

No one would deny that the Wolf has a sex drive and, for purpose of argument, let us assume that it is stronger than average (setting aside the real possibility that he may doubt his virility). If his goal were to maximize his opportunity for sexual relations, he could achieve it by marrying and settling down to what George Bernard Shaw once called "the most licentious of human institutions." [1] Frequent sexual experience is more readily achieved in marriage than in an intermittent succession of affairs. In fact, most of the Wolf's married acquaintances copulate more times in a year than he does.

If this point is brought to his attention, the Wolf answers that he seeks variety as well as frequency of sexual experience. At this point, however, he is no longer arguing on the basis of his physiological need. The sexual drive *per se* merely motivates the individual toward sexual activity, and there is no physiological reason why an assortment of partners should be preferred.

Admittedly, man is a primate, and it does seem to be the nature of many primates to copulate with most other primates they encounter. But man is also a creature of habit. He could sit with anyone when he enters a bar, but he looks around for a familiar face. American culture permits promiscuity in choice of dinner companions, but he usually eats at the same place with the same people. If the culture were as permissive about sexual promiscuity, the odds are that the average American would have intercourse with someone other than his wife about as often as he chooses to eat out.

The Wolf's desire for constant variety in sexual partners is primarily a rationalization of his desire to keep his relations with women transitory. He does not want to become "entangled." That is to say, he seeks only superficial relationships because he is afraid of close association. Marriage is threatening to him not primarily because of the restraints it might impose, but because of the intimacy it would entail.

Like many of his fellows, the Wolf hides behind a role which he plays well. By being a Wolf, he conceals himself; besides, he doubts that *he* is acceptable, but he has some confidence in his ability to play the role of the seducer. The successes of years (and a knowledge of what prospects to abandon early in the game) have given him assurance. Moreover, if some sweet young thing spurns his advances, he can assume that her behavior reflects her inhibitions, not his unacceptability.

The Wolf tries to substitute physical intimacy for intimate association. His understanding of close relationships has changed surprisingly little since his childhood, and he interprets his need to be with others as a desire to return to the warmth and comfort he knew in his mother's arms. But he is a product of a culture that does not regard wanting to be cuddled and comforted as manly. His desire to be cuddled thus seems to threaten his self-image as a virile male, and so he transmutes it into sexual desire.

He is preoccupied with the female breast. The first thing he notices in a woman are her mammaries, and they are a focal point of his sex play. This interest seems so naturally sexual to the American that he never wonders about it. Yet the breasts have no physical function in the act of coitus—they are one erogenous zone among many. Most Americans are surprised to learn that the breast is not a sexual object in many societies, including the famous barebreasted cultures of the South Seas. Biologically, it would be as logical to be excited by small feet as by large breasts, and in traditional Chinese culture the former fascination was as normal as the latter is in American culture. (Note that in both cultures nature was abandoned in favor of artifice: Chinese foot binding and the American uplift brassière.)

But preoccupation with the breast does involve more than merely a culturally defined interest. The breast may lack a function in coitus, but it has a biological function: to feed and soothe the child. The Wolf has a strong tendency to value the breast for this very reason. He sees it as a symbol of comfort and security.

Yet he could not imagine saying to a woman, "I want to fondle your breasts because I feel insecure." An admission of his desire to be comforted would seem threatening to him (unless he rationalized it as part of a seductive "line"). But he can say, "Your breasts excite me." This seems virile—and safe. It keeps the relationship in the sexual realm where his role shields him from the revealing intimacy he fears.

Moreover, he is likely to be quite hostile to women. They may be the symbol of comfort withheld. Somewhere in the childhood of the Wolf lies deep and bitter conflict with his mother or some other emotionally significant woman—at least he has never learned to interact with women as people, only as sexual objects. His affairs are thus impersonal and marked by aggressive sexual behavior. (In this he carries to an extreme behavior what is not uncommon among American males. The very slang employed to describe seduction and impregnation indicates the hostile, coercive overtones in normal American sexual behavior —"to make," "to screw," "to knock up.")

Thus the Wolf's relations with women are deliberately impersonal and more than a little hostile. He is not likely to find fulfillment of his need for intimate association in the pseudo-intimacy of his transitory affairs. His friendships with men are rare, in part because he spends his time pursuing women, in part because many of the women he seduces are the employees or wives of men he knows, but above all because with men he cannot establish the physical intimacy which is the only form of intimacy he permits himself.

Attempting to substitute sexual intimacy for intimate association, seeking indirect self-acceptance by playing a successful sexual role with women and bragging about his success to men, he diverts his energies from the unfilled needs which motivate him. For all his brave show of seductive charm, the Wolf remains needful, uncertain, and lonely.

The Girl Who Can't Say No

The promiscuous girl has somewhat different motivations from the Wolf, or at least a different view of herself and her behavior. As she sees herself, she merely succumbs to her sexual desires, but at the same time she often acknowledges that she derives rather little enjoyment from sex. The physiological sexual drive accounts for her behavior no more than it does for that of the Wolf.

Typically, such a girl feels inadequate in comparison to other girls, believing that they have some inexplicable femininity, some attractive quality that she lacks. She thinks the only way she can be attractive to men is to offer intercourse. Through a succession of affairs she seeks the intimate association she craves and assurance that she is an adequate, attractive woman.

Her major concern is rarely fear of pregnancy, but rather fear that persons who are emotionally significant to her (usually her parents) will discover her sexual activity. Indeed, she is likely to be surprisingly careless about pregnancy, a carelessness which suggests an underlying desire to confront others with unquestionable proof of her sexual activity and adequacy. Such a desire is in fact usually part of her motivation.

Consciously she may fear being discovered and be concerned that her actions might hurt others. But the unrecognized side of her ambivalence is a desire to defy and to hurt. Promiscuity is the most obvious and extreme form of rebellion for the young girl in American culture—and the easiest. It takes little initiative on her part, and she can rationalize her behavior by claiming an uncontrollable sexual drive.

The adventuring wife has similar motivations. With each affair she seeks to prove her adequacy as a woman and to hurt her husband. She may believe that the intimacy of marriage has revealed her shortcomings to her husband and that he has lost interest in her. (Such a wife will be considered at length in chapter 10.)

The adulterous wife seeks indirect self-acceptance from paramours, who are quite willing to assure her that she is witty, charming, and sexually exciting after thirty. But she suspects their motivation and suspects also that her desirability is largely a matter of

availability. To ease her misgivings she may rationalize her behavior as retaliation against her husband for
some grievance (she may tell herself that this is rec-
ompense for his hostile, aggressive lovemaking, or for
his infidelities). Or she may rationalize it by assuming that she has an unusually intense sexual drive. Her
self-doubts are not diminished either way.

The Jealous Wife

Extreme promiscuity is the exception among American women, most of whom sexualize their needs to
some degree but respond to the sexualization in an
inhibited fashion. A frequent pattern is to project
the sexualized desire and to become preoccupied with
the presumed sexual interests of others. This pattern
characterizes the wife who fears her (as yet) faithful
husband's desires for extramarital adventure. Whenever another woman is present, this jealous wife
watches her closely. She also watches her husband
and is practically certain that he is wondering what
this other woman would be like in bed. Her associations with other women are strained, for she evaluates
each as a potential sexual rival.

When she upbraids her husband for his roving eye,
she points out that she has been a faithful wife in
thought as well as in deed—and not for lack of opportunity. She is convinced that most of the men she
meets desire her, and keeping men at a safe distance
is an additional source of anxiety to her. The poor
woman thus finds her relations with both sexes vastly
complicated by the sexual interests she imputes to
others.

For the sake of argument, let us assume that she is
often quite correct in her assumptions about what her
husband and other men are thinking (although there
is some question about the number of men that would

undertake seducing someone as stiff and inhibited as she is). Even so, her indignant response reveals her own projected thoughts. Her preoccupation with sex arises from a number of fears and confusions. She is likely to have difficulty accepting and acting on her sexual desires, a difficulty which leads her to give a sexual focus to her general fears of inadequacy. Moreover, she is likely to sexualize her need for intimate association. Having given her needs for self-acceptance and association a sexual cast, she magnifies her sexual drive and it seems a compelling desire. Certain that such a desire is not suitable for a lady she alienates and projects her lascivious thoughts and blushes at what some man is thinking.

The Hidden Fear

By no means all sexualization involves relations between the sexes; on the contrary, the sexualization people fear most in themselves is of a different type. Imagine a man who has been riding an interstate bus for many miles. His head is propped on the corner of the seat next to his as he sprawls in sleep. The bus makes a brief stop and a new passenger boards. He sits down next to the dozing traveler, and the latter pulls himself sharply over against the window, well away from his new companion. Although he attempts to resume his nap, he shifts uneasily about in his seat, visibly uncomfortable in the situation. Why?

The man has been traveling alone for many hours and is wanting companionship. The new passenger offers him an opportunity. He feels a vague desire to talk to the man, to seek the pleasure of association. He even has a fleeting awareness of an urge to express warmth physically, perhaps to rest his head on the man's shoulder. But in American culture such a desire is considered appropriate only for children or lovers.

Not being a child, he assumes that the wish indicates a desire for sexual intimacy. Thus he sexualizes a desire for bodily contact which is in reality no more sexual than the nuzzling of a puppy. The natural inclination of a lonely man seems to him a frightening symptom of homosexuality.

The American male can endure many insults and admit many shortcomings, but call him homosexual and he is likely to become violent. Thus the traveler is secretly frightened and openly annoyed as he turns to the window silently cursing because he no longer has the seat to himself. He remains lonely and needful and the resulting tensions aggravate his discomfort.

Similar scenes are repeated countless times each day. American men place many restraints on warm association with each other, largely because they sexualize their need for intimate association with their own sex. These sexualized desires are feared and alienated and then projected onto the homosexual (which is the basic reason why he is so widely loathed). The reverse side of the confusion is a common element in homosexuality: the individual affirms such sexualization and becomes preoccupied with it.

Yet the underlying need is merely for warm, candid association. The sexualization of this need complicates a man's relations with half of the people he knows. And his relations with the feminine half are complicated by more-overt sexualizations.

Confusion is sometimes compounded. Consider the man who allows himself to lower his defenses only in the secure atmosphere of a particular friendship. When he is with this friend he enjoys warm association, but he also experiences a desire for bodily contact which frightens him. Such contact is a natural expression of friendly warmth, as any group of uninhibited children at play will demonstrate. But in America any physical contact between men is tabu— unless it is a handshake, a punch in the arm, or a slap on the back. So fear enters the relationship.

At last the man rationalizes his physical attraction by transferring it to his friend's wife. This, too, is a forbidden desire but at least it does not pose a threat to his conception of manhood. He is ashamed to think about making advances to the wife of his best friend, but he is able to believe that "falling in love" was not his fault.

In the long run he is likely to lose his friend one way or another. He may become an open rival, or he may become so uncomfortable about the situation that he avoids both his friend and his friend's wife. The sexualization and the resulting misinterpretations lead him far from his original need and cost him a rewarding friendship.

Women seem to be less prone to this form of sexualization than men. Perhaps this is because there are fewer restrictions on physical contact between women in American culture. A woman can literally cry on her friend's shoulder, or kiss her in greeting, without violating cultural tabus. If a woman becomes attracted to her best friend's husband it is not usually because she fears a sexual attachment to her friend. More often, she feels inadequate in comparison to her friend and by seducing the husband hopes to prove herself as desirable as the woman she admires.

Sex

Sexual desire (as distinct from sexualized desires) is a physiologically based drive which can afford considerable physical pleasure and/or result in conception, and that is all that it is. Sexual situations do offer opportunities for the simultaneous satisfaction of certain other needs, notably the need for intimate association. Approached in these terms, sexual activity can result in both physical and psychic satisfaction.

But it is one thing to satisfy needs simultaneously and quite another to try to substitute satisfaction of one need for another. When the self needs are sexualized the individual attempts to utilize sex as a means of indirect self-acceptance, of disguised aggression, as a substitute for intimate association, as a means of rebellion—and the sexual enjoyment is impaired while the other needs involved remain deprived. Out of such neurotic confusions arise most of the "sexual" problems in American culture.

9
INTIMACY

I still find that some people imagine that intimacy is only a matter of approximating genitals one to another. . . . Intimacy . . . requires a type of relationship which I call collaboration, by which I mean clearly formulated adjustments of one's behavior to the expressed needs of the other person in the pursuit of increasingly identical—that is, more and more nearly mutual—satisfactions. HARRY STACK SULLIVAN

Despite the barriers he normally erects between himself and others, the adjusted American allows himself a few intimate associations. Yet, even in these relationships, he is dogged by normal neurosis. In chapter 3 we discussed three aspects of the need for association: the need for others as mirrors, as models, and as the recipients of actions. All three aspects are commonly complicated by misinterpretations and misdirection.

The Mutual Admiration Society

In his neurotic quest for indirect self-acceptance, the adjusted American usually seeks a flattering mirror—not an honest one. Even intimate association may be turned to this dubious end, a pattern which can be seen in exaggerated form among adolescent girls. Girls of thirteen or fourteen, engaged in an intense search for their womanhood, try on new gestures, opinions, and figures of speech for much the same reason that they try on new clothes. The girl poses before her mirror—and before her best friend—asking, "How do I look?" or "What am I like?" But she is more interested in enthusiastic approval than in an honest answer.

In their interminable telephone conversations one details her thoughts and feelings and recapitulates her actions while the other clucks sympathy and approval; then they trade roles. What one thinks of a hair style, a dress, a boy friend, or an idea is the overriding influence on the other—much to the annoyance of their respective parents. Each takes note of any compliments paid the other (often soliciting them) and trades for compliments which the other has collected about her. The screams and giggles which accompany these exchanges indicate the importance the girls attach to such bits of flattery.

In short, these girls have a mutual admiration society, each trading her approval and support for the other's. A second tie between them is a nonaggression pact, a commitment to do nothing to hurt or to embarrass each other. (If it is violated, the friendship will in all probability dissolve acrimoniously.) This aspect of the relationship precludes any blunt observation that might lead to hurt feelings, and in practice it also rules out the candor which could enable each girl to refine and verify her self-image.

Such mutual admiration societies and nonaggression pacts are common (if usually more subtle) in adult friendships. There is a tacit agreement that one person will believe another is likable and admirable provided that the other reciprocates. Without making it explicit, most Americans regard such an arrangement as basic to friendship.

In effect, such pacts represent an attempt to make

indirect self-acceptance work. But like all other efforts to achieve self-acceptance indirectly they founder on inherent contradictions. The party to a mutual admiration society inevitably discounts the image of himself which is reflected in the flattering attitudes of the other. However much he wants to believe the gratifying image his friend holds up, he knows that it is payment in kind. He cannot quite give it credence.

There is nothing inherently misdirected in a non-aggression pact. Indeed, if most people did not operate largely on the basis of such tacit understandings, society would disintegrate into Hobbes's conception of the war of each against all. But when any honest criticism is regarded as hostile attack, a nonaggression pact renders association a tissue of flattering half-truths. Sooner or later one party to it is likely to weary of guarding his words and buoying up the other's spirits, especially if he feels he is giving more support than he is receiving. At this point he is likely to make critical comments that *are* barbed and the friendship shatters. Perhaps it is no great loss.

Intimacy based on mutual admiration and nonaggression pacts serves more as a palliative for feelings of inadequacy than as a means of developing self-acceptance. The parties to a mutual admiration society may feel dependent on each other, but they do not necessarily enjoy each other. Note that while the adolescent girls may be miserable apart, they are often bored and listless when together.

Reciprocal Rationalization

Another variation on the distorted mirror effect is the attempt to seek out people who will reflect one's failings or problems from a favorable angle because they share them. Thus the fanatic who refuses insight because he fears it might lead him to abandon his biases welcomes another fanatic who will assert that he is not biased at all. Or two rebels may be drawn to each other because each is able to justify the other's rebellion. They discuss at length the failure of others (parents, or perhaps current spouses) to understand them: i.e., failure to give dignity to their rebellious behavior. The rebels may come to feel a profound desire to be together and many an unsuccesful marriage has been based on such a relationship. (A partner in rebellion seldom makes a satisfactory marriage partner—the rebels soon begin to rebel against each other, or one outgrows the rebellion.)

It is not difficult to determine when reciprocal rationalization lies at the core of a relationship. Each person feels drawn to the other, wants to be with him, yet is almost always a little tense with him. The tension reveals the nature of the association. Each is drawn to the other because he is trying *to justify behaviors or beliefs about which he is extremely dubious*. If he were not dubious, he would not be going to such lengths to rationalize and dignify his behavior.

Thus the common bond is something about which both are uncomfortable at the outset and the interaction between them serves to focus their attention on it. They may try to rationalize their tension by such convenient explanations as "If only we were free we could escape this sense of furtiveness. . . ." But if they were free the discomfort would remain; a misdirection does not become rewarding merely because two people pursue it together.

Reciprocal rationalization is one basis of the phenomenon called counter-transference in which a psychotherapist feels an intense attraction to his patient. A therapist often comes to feel that he should not have any unresolved problems. Encountering a patient who shows problems similar to ones which he himself has failed to resolve, the therapist may project his own alienated problems onto the patient. Thus he explains them away and at the same time is able to justify and dignify them. He is likely to see this patient as an appealing and tragic figure, caught up in inner conflicts which are very difficult to resolve and somehow noble. He and the patient share and rationalize the problem, and the prognosis for this therapy is poor indeed.

The intimacy found in a mutual admiration society or derived from reciprocal rationalization is marred by attempts to persuade others to reflect a distorted image of the self. Such misdirection blocks the fulfillment of the first aspect of the need for association: the need for others as accurate mirrors.

Unrecognized Self-Discovery

Almost inevitably other people serve as models for the individual, but misdirection or misinterpretation may prevent them from being useful models. It frequently happens that a person develops capacities similar to those he admires in others without being aware of the process. He may explore and enjoy unsuspected facets of himself without recognizing them as his own.

Picture a shy girl who has lived several years in a large city without making more than the most casual acquaintances. Timid and uncertain of herself, she seeks the apparent safety of the known, building a routine existence that moves in a narrow pattern from boardinghouse to office to movie theater and back to boardinghouse. She longs for friends but so restricts herself that she fades into the background and is overlooked by others. She waits for someone to take the initiative and for a long time she waits in vain.

Suppose this girl acquires a roommate with an unusual capacity for enjoying life. Her own life is suddenly transformed. Following her new friend's enthusiasms, she finds herself playing tennis, sailing, learning the newest dance steps, exploring the restaurants, shops, galleries, and theaters of the city. Where before she perceived only drab uniformity she now finds drama and color—in the city, in other people—above all in herself.

One of the unquestioned assumptions of American culture is the belief that emotions have an external explanation. When an American feels angry he looks around to see what provoked him, and when he feels happy he looks around to see who delighted him. Conforming unwittingly to this assumption, this girl believes that her new roommate is making her happy. This is only indirectly true. Her friend is the catalyst but the changes are within herself. Her happiness results from the discovery and development of her own capacities. Taking her friend as a model she has explored unsuspected dimensions of her self.

Her self-discovery goes unrecognized, however. She knows that her life was dull before her friend moved in, her life is now exciting, and she assumes therefore that her friend is the cause of her new-found joy in living. *Post hoc, ergo propter hoc*, the most common fallacy known to man.

To insist that the roommate was only indirectly the cause of her pleasure may seem to split hairs. However, the consequences of confusion on the point can be real and painful. Believing that her friend is the source of her enjoyment, the girl is more concerned with trying to monopolize her than with imitating her example. Without intending it, she encourages her friend to seek other, less-demanding companions. Thus the shy girl's pleasure may dissolve in bitter jealousy. The full consequences of the misinterpretation appear if her roommate moves out. The girl will mourn her loss and slip back into her old withdrawn and restricted pattern, unaware that the girl she had found most exciting was herself.

Intimate association which involves *unrecognized* self-discovery may be stimulating while it lasts, but it contains within itself the seeds of discord. (If the self-discovery is conscious that is quite another matter. Conscious self-discovery through association is a highly rewarding and direct avenue to self-acceptance.) The person who does not recognize the inner source of his delight clings possessively to his friend and fails to revise his self-image to include his nascent capacities.

Restricted Warmth

A familiar dramatic plot involves a broken, withdrawn man who becomes responsible for a needful child and in caring for the child finds himself and becomes whole again. There is considerable insight in this theme. Many aspects of the self which the individual values can be experienced only through actions toward others. A man cannot be warm, understanding, kind, loyal, and many other things which the adjusted American has learned to want to be unless there is someone *to whom* he can be these things. He needs a recipient for his actions in order to act on his potential, and unless he acts on it he can derive no satisfaction from it nor can it form a viable part of his self-image.

The adjusted American restricts his opportunities to experience his warm, outgoing potential. In part this is because he maintains defenses which inhibit the expression of warmth (as discussed at length in chapter 7). But in part, too, he deprives himself of countless opportunities to experience his own warmth because he assumes that it must be elicited by others. He assumes his warm feelings are called forth in response to some quality in his most intimate associates, and he does not perceive that warmth is a capacity within himself that he can act on at will with almost anyone as the recipient.

The result is that he has fewer intimate associates than he could have, and he forfeits the pleasure he could find in being warm toward casual acquaintances. Part of the popularity of Christmas is the custom of being warm toward everyone as part of the "holiday spirit." What a pity that American culture only encourages this two or three weeks a year!

Localized Self-Acceptance

The most rewarding intimacy is that in which all three aspects of the need for association are fulfilled. The adjusted American may have one or two friends and perhaps a spouse with whom he feels free to let down the walls and to relax the restraints he imposes on himself in other association. In the company of such a friend he drops his roles and can smile at revealing slips. Making no effort at pretense, he feels accepted for what he is—faults included. His relief at being able to lower his defenses, coupled with his relief that what he reveals is not held against him, leads him to feel profoundly comfortable. He lets his friend be a mirror—an honest mirror—and discovers that, taken all in all, he likes what he sees.

Such a friend is likely also to be a model. An association in which the individual feels free to drop his pretenses is also one in which he feels comfortable about imitating the capacities he admires in his friend. If a skill is involved, he may ask his friend to teach him; if what he admires is an attitude toward life, he tries it out to see if it suits him, with his friend present to set the tone. The result is conscious and rewarding self-discovery.

In actions toward his friend, the individual expresses capacities which he values, and is thus able to verify the inclusion of such capacities in his self-image. Expecting to feel warm and sympathetic toward his friend, he does. He recognizes and acts on the opportunity to be an amusing companion, a trusted confidant, a willing partner in adventure.

The ties between such friends are habits of mutual need satisfaction. Such habits include, but go far beyond, the simple reciprocity implied in the folk expression "I'll scratch your back, you scratch mine." Mutual need satisfaction results from interaction in which each serves as a mirror for the other, helping him to refine his self-image and to evaluate himself; each expands his self-image and develops self-potential, taking his friend as a model; each is the recipient of actions through which the other verifies a valued self-image. Each is helped to achieve an accurate and acceptable self-image—self-acceptance—in association with the other.

However, the adjusted American is seldom able to achieve such self-acceptance in other situations, outside the protective environment of a close friendship. Such self-acceptance as he achieves, therefore, tends to be *localized*.

Nevertheless, localized self-acceptance is fundamentally different from indirect self-acceptance. Localized self-acceptance can be achieved, but indirect self-acceptance is an unattainable delusion. The person engaged in the neurotic quest for indirect self-acceptance tries to put forward only those qualities which he feels are beyond reproach and tries to conceal from others a self which he fears is unacceptable. In contrast, the person able to experience localized self-acceptance is presenting himself openly and candidly to his friend and is able to give credence to his reflection in the eyes of the other. In the relationship his virtues seem more accessible and his faults less damning. *Localized self-acceptance is direct self-acceptance, experienced sporadically under favorable circumstances.*

Localized self-acceptance lies behind the phenomenon of transference in psychotherapy. In the shelter and security of the office, the patient ultimately reveals his fears and secrets. When he discovers that honesty does not impair his warm relation to the therapist, he finds an ideal environment for self-acceptance. The resulting sense of fulfillment is exhilarating, and the patient gratefully attributes it to the therapist. In successful psychotherapy, the patient gradually learns to carry his self-acceptance (and the modes of interaction which facilitate it) outside the sheltered confines of the consulting room.

Transference is not unique to psychotherapy. The person who achieves localized self-acceptance in any rewarding association is likely to attribute his enjoyment to his friend's warmth, broadminded acceptance, sense of humor, or simply to the experiences he and his friend have shared. Yet the enjoyment he derives in the association is influenced far more by *how* he associates than by with *whom* he associates.

Believing that his friend elicits the sense of well-being he enjoys, he misses the importance of his own behavior. His assumption that the good feeling is caused by his friend leads to particularization: the equation of a particular means of satisfaction with the need itself. When feeling depressed and inadequate, he thinks he needs his friend. If his friend is not present, he remains deprived. Thus the limitation of localized self-acceptance is that the continuing need for self-acceptance is satisfied only sporadically.

Bereavement

If a person finds self-acceptance only within a particular relationship, he has a tremendous stake in that relationship. If he loses the friend, spouse, or parent with whom he found localized self-acceptance, he suffers severe deprivation. (This idea is expressed with poignant humor in the quip "Mother loved me, but she died.")

When the loss is through death, special problems ensue. Imagine a woman confronted with the sudden death of her husband after a quarter of a century of marriage. The marriage had been successful: that is, the couple had developed many habits of mutual need satisfaction which bound them together. Their closeness had involved localized self-acceptance, for in the microcosm of a rewarding marriage there was no reason for (nor possibility of) the pretenses they maintained with outsiders. The relationship had been functional and satisfying to a considerable degree, but highly particularized. Each had believed that the other "made" him happy.

With her husband's death, the woman experiences a vast loss. She has lost her husband and with him her habitual modes of need satisfaction. The localized self-acceptance she found within her marriage has been cut short and her self-acceptance falters. Mounting deprivation creates a state of extreme tension—a state which she has learned to interpret as anger. And she assumes that someone must have made her angry.

This misinterpretation leads her to conclude that she is angry at her husband for dying. She recoils from this idea the moment it crosses her mind (if indeed she lets it rise to consciousness at all). She regards the idea as monstrous. She knows that her husband did not want to die, and she knows that her anger is unjustified. But her tense needfulness remains. Unable to recognize it as deprivation and unwilling to regard it as anger, she turns it back against herself as grief.

This pattern is normal in American culture (and in many others). The death of someone close to the individual disrupts the familiar patterns of need satisfaction and deprives the survivor. The bereaved individual tends to interpret the tension which accompanies need as anger—anger at the one who died. But because such anger is tabu, the individual disguises it. He may transfer it to someone else—perhaps to a relative who cannot wait for the will to be read or to a hospital which seemed to provide inadequate care. But mostly he will turn it against himself as grief and despair. At this point he typically withdraws from life (at least for a time), precisely at the moment when he is most needful.

The Scope of Intimacy

The adjusted American has learned to expect intimacy only in exceptional friendships. He thus finds it only occasionally. The rest of his association is reduced to role playing in which he seeks to conceal much of himself. Even much of his intimate association is twisted toward misdirected ends as he seeks a supportive relationship rather than the open, candid relationship which could contribute to insight and self-acceptance.

He has been encouraged by his culture to devote far more attention to searching for rewarding companions than to developing rewarding modes of interaction. Thus instead of learning to satisfy his needs continually among the people he happens to be with, he pulls back within his walls except when he is with particular friends. Undeniably, some people are more stimulating companions than others. But the person who withholds himself from most people ends by depriving himself most of the time.

10
LOVE OR MARRIAGE

Why, you would not make a man your lawyer or your family doctor on so slight an acquaintance as you would fall in love with and marry him!

GEORGE BERNARD SHAW

The typical American really believes that it is impossible to understand why he falls in love. He does, however, have a clear idea of how to tell *when* he is in love: he expects to be at once ecstatic and miserable, to behave erratically, to experience a floating sensation, and to lose his appetite. Sophisticated Americans discount these notions, but not as much as they think they do. They smile at romantic love but expound earnestly on "real love" or "mature love." They debate the merits of different forms of love, but never seem to question the idea of love itself.

The American divorce rate has been variously attributed to teenage marriage, delayed marriage, premarital sexual experience, lack of sexual experience, decline of religious influence, residual Puritanism, glamorization of divorce, and even the automobile. But our analysis suggests a different, perhaps a shocking answer: American marriages are unstable because Americans marry for love.

Let it be understood at the outset that we are not confining our discussion to the romantic notions of adolescents, suggesting that all would be well if only they achieved "mature love." It is love itself, mature or immature, real or illusory, which we are challenging.

Because the myth of love is deeply imbedded in American culture, such an assertion may seem absurd, even threatening. The American fears that his life (and especially his marriage) would be flat and joyless without love. Moreover, he thinks that without someone to love him he could never accept himself.

Yet the questioning of any widely accepted myth seems initially unsettling. It was once feared that if people lost faith in the proposition that kings ruled by Divine Right, no authority would be tolerated and anarchy would engulf society. And once a myth is dead, it seems incredible that anyone ever took it seriously.

By no means do all peoples take love seriously. There are societies in which love is regarded as a rare form of insanity. There are other societies which have no word for love except as a euphemism for sexual desire. There are still other societies which speak simply of sexual desire, and have no word for love in their language.

When the adjusted American learns that love is not universal, he is likely to express pity (if not contempt) for people who are so backward or so cold that they do not fall in love. He has been imbued with the notion that love is of supreme importance in life, and he considers any adult who has never been in love to be emotionally stunted.

This belief in the power of love to transform and to mature the individual is curiously parallel to the aboriginal American Indian belief in the power of trance experience. It was the custom in many tribes to send adolescent boys into the hills in search of a vision. To some a vision came easily and soon; to others it came only after days of fasting. But, until it came, a boy could not become a man. His vision endowed him with power for life, and determined whether he would become a hunter, warrior, shaman, or transvestite.

The American would be amused at the suggestion that he choose his career while in a trance, as the Indian boy did. Yet he finds nothing odd in the practices of choosing a wife according to the vagaries of the ecstatic trance he calls love. Ethnocentrism aside, the one practice is as illogical as the other.

But the American takes for granted the view of love which is inculcated by his culture. The only question he is prepared to raise about love regards its authenticity: is his feeling infatuation or is it the Real Thing? Circumstances which might lead an objective observer to have grave doubts about a marriage seem insignificant to the American in love. It is an article of faith with him that love conquers all. *His question is not whether the marriage would be sound, but whether his love is real.*

If concern about the authenticity of an ecstatic experience has a medieval ring, it might be recalled that romantic love is an invention of the Middle Ages. The troubadours built the myth of love and fashioned such ideas as love at first sight, the existence of an Ideal lover for each person, and the power of True Love to conquer all. One glimpse of the fair maiden leaning over the parapet and the knight was supposed to be smitten. He might pine away if his love was not returned, but let his lady encourage him by some token and his strength was increased tenfold. Possessed by love, he had the power to conquer all obstacles in his path, including any dragons guarding the maiden.

But in the Middle Ages love was not the basis for

marriage. Family connections, land ownership, political convenience, and at times even military alliance were the foundations of aristocratic marriage. And peasant marriages were contracted on similarly pragmatic bases. Romantic love was an aristocratic diversion, but the nobility that amused itself with love explicitly assumed that love and marriage were incompatible. The daily familiarities of marriage could only erode romance. So it was not his bride that the medieval prince expected to love, modern fairy tales to the contrary notwithstanding; when knighthood was in flower, one knight's love was another knight's lady.

At the end of the Middle Ages, the emerging middle class adopted the aristocratic ideology of love. But the middle class was uncomfortable about the extramarital setting, so they made love fit their moral code. Keeping the medieval idea of love nearly intact, they wrapped it into a neat middle-class package by making love the basis for marriage. As individual choice gradually superseded family dictates, marriage for love became part of Western tradition.

And so Americans marry for love—a culturally defined emotion which was considered incompatible with marriage by those who shaped it. Americans regard as a supreme experience an emotional seizure which some peoples consider akin to running amuck. They deliberately place love beyond comprehension and control, and thereby surrender in advance any hope of autonomous choice when love affects their lives. And then—wondrous irony—they demand to know what has gone wrong with their marriages.

Love can be fun, and the autonomous individual might choose to experience it—but hardly as a basis for marriage. Choosing a spouse while under the influence of an emotion which the individual himself insists is unpredictable, incomprehensible, and irresistible is incompatible with autonomy. One could as well marry while drunk. But fortunately love *is* comprehensible and (to a surprising degree) predictable. And, once understood, love need not be a compulsive emotion.

This Thing Called Love

A love affair may involve many of the mechanisms found in friendship: a mutual admiration society, a nonaggression pact, unrecognized self-discovery, reciprocal rationalization, habits of mutual need satisfaction—all of these, or none. But the unique quality of love itself derives from yet a different psychological mechanism. Love *is* more than friendship.

Men love much as they hate; the mechanism of the one emotion is an inversion of the other. When a person alienates from himself some quality or potential which he despises, he projects it onto someone else, where he hates it. Conversely, when he alienates some quality or potential which he would like to experience in himself but does not, he projects it onto someone else, where he loves it. The people he loves, like those he hates, are merely convenient targets for his projections.

It may seem curious that anyone would alienate potentialities he longs to experience in himself, but there are several reasons why people do so. Often, the individual alienates qualities that seem contradictory to his fundamental self-image. He may regard these characteristics as desirable in abstract, but as inappropriate for himself. Thus he may not permit himself reckless bravado, impulsiveness, impracticality, whimsey, or bounding optimism, but he may project his potential for such behaviors onto someone else and adore it in them. Here lies the reason for the attraction of opposites (although lovers may not seem so opposite to outsiders as they seem to each other).

Many of the characteristics which are alienated from the self and loved in others are those which the culture has assigned to the opposite sex. Most societies designate some behaviors and qualities as "masculine" and others as "feminine." But this does not mean that men are devoid of potential normally attributed to women, or vice versa. On the contrary, what is normal masculine behavior in one culture may be normal feminine behavior in another. Margaret Mead reports that among the Tchambuli of New Guinea the women are expected to be practical, comradely, and sexually aggresive, whereas the men are expected to be passive and artistic, to gossip and primp.[1] For that matter, not far back in Western history the dashing cavalier wore long curls and perfume; with the rapier and stallion went powder and lace and soft leather boots that displayed a well-turned calf. Whatever is defined as "manly" at a given time and place determines to a large degree which of his potentialities a boy will try to realize and which he will alienate.

In modern America, boys past the age of four or five learn that it is not manly to cry, to want to be cuddled, to be fearful, too clean, or too pretty. Although the boy may enjoy indulging some of these characteristics (such as his desire to be cuddled), he comes to disown them as he seeks to become an acceptable man. As his self-image is directed toward the cultural image of masculinity, he alienates his potential for responding in "feminine" ways.

This alienation does not rid him either of his capacity for responding in these ways, or of his potential enjoyment of such responses. He would still like to be cuddled and fussed over, to be comforted when hurt, to adorn himself. But the stronger side of his ambivalence is the desire to be a little reserved, rugged, and "masculine" in appearance and demeanor, to shrug aside offers of condolence. A man coming out of anesthesia once summarized the ambivalence by growling at his wife "Go away and stop leaving me alone!"

Having alienated those aspects of himself which he has learned to regard as incompatible with his manhood, the male projects them onto the women around him. In his mother, his daughter, his wife, and particularly his sweetheart, he sees and loves his own desires to be dependent, vain, impractical, demonstrative, and all the other things he has learned to consider unsuitable in himself. Indeed, he often demands that his women display such characteristics.

In a parallel but reverse manner, the little girl in America is encouraged to seek comfort when she scrapes a knee, to be openly affectionate, to be proud of her curls and ruffles—and is scolded for a dirty face or a bold manner. She learns to alienate her potential for being aggressive, self-assertive, proficient in sports and mechanics. She is likely to adore masterful men.

It would be oversimplification to view the cultural ideal for men and for women as direct opposites, corresponding like a photographic print to its negative. But there are many qualities which one sex is encouraged to display and the other to alienate and project. These customary projections on the opposite sex lead to a general attraction of men to women and vice versa—over and above the biological interest in the opposite sex.

Another reason for alienating and projecting valued facets of the self is that a person may become falsely convinced that he lacks some quality which he considers desirable. As a child he may have been reminded of his inability to do something so often that the deficiency became an established part of his self-image. As his parents dwelt on the capacity, they underscored its desirability at the same time that they convinced the child that he lacked it. However great or small his potential in this area might have been, the child came to cherish it at the same time that he alienated it. His capacity may remain inaccessible to him throughout his life. If so, he will experience it only via projection on others—to whom he feels strongly attracted.

Having always been told, say, that he has no talent for making friends (but like anyone else having some ability to do so) he alienates his potential and projects it onto someone who displays an outgoing, gregarious nature. He will then find himself drawn to this person, perhaps (if other projections follow the first) "falling in love." But the love is for lost facets of himself. Almost everyone has a minimal capacity to do almost anything humanly possible—and the person who is in fact totally deficient in some quality is not likely to value it in others. He may be aware of qualities which he lacks, but he will not adore them: the color-blind man is not enamored of the artist's color sense. The qualities he adores in others are his own displaced potentialities.

Thus each individual makes idiosyncratic alienations which fill in details on the cultural image of the opposite sex, and out of these he creates his own specific "Ideal." The subsequent search for the Ideal mate is in reality a quest for the alienated but desired facets of the self which have been shaped into the idealized image. When a man first falls in love he simply hangs this image on some woman and loves it. If the fit is extremely poor, he may soon withdraw his projections—and believe that he was only "infatuated." But if the ready-made image fits her reasonably well (with a few alterations in minor details) and if other positive projections supplement those of the original ideal image, he is soon a man in love.

Bystanders (who are not making comparable projections) may wonder what he sees in her, or shrug and say that love is blind. In a sense it is, for the lover peers through a haze of projections. Even if the projections are a good fit, it does not alter the fact that it is his own alienated potential that he loves. The compelling power of love derives from the desire to reunite with the alienated and loved capacities of the self.

The adolescent girl who sighs and screams over a singer she has never seen off the stage is ridiculed by her elders, but she is correct in insisting that she is in love. Her emotion is love in its purest form; that is, it is not an admixture of romance and friendship. Her love is, moreover, in the best medieval tradition; inaccessibility of the beloved was originally a vital element in romantic love. Distance enables the lover to see his beloved purely in terms of the projections he hangs on her.

The demonstration that love is not caused by unique qualities of the beloved is as simple as noting that a constant cannot explain a variable. John may not love Mary, may come to love Mary, and may cease to love Mary—all while Mary remains unchanged. Clearly it is something within the lover which causes him to love, and that something is the desire to recapture alienated self-potential. Beauty is in the eye of the beholder, as the saying goes, and so is love.

The True Love of John and Mary

John has definite ideas about what he wants in a wife. To the cultural expectation that she must be exciting, warm, pretty, dainty, and in need of his love and protection, he has added various other potentialities which through circumstance he has alienated from his self-image. All he needs is a target on which he can project this idealized image—and Mary dances by. He hears her laugh, and feels a sudden "irresistible attraction." He flings after his impression of a girl the image that he is prepared to love, and is drawn to it. The basic mechanism would have been the same had he fallen gradually in love with the girl next door, but John happens to fall in love at first sight. He maneuvers an introduction, and the romance begins.

A romance is a prime situation in which to enjoy many aspects of the self. It offers an opportunity for being loving and lovable, excited and exciting. It puts John in a mood to enjoy himself, even under circumstances (such as waiting for a bus in the rain) that he would normally have thought miserable. He surprises himself with the ingenuity he uses to find places to take Mary, and things to do. By tradition (and because parties to a romance are usually at a stage in life when other responsibilities are not too burdensome) many pleasant activities are virtually set aside for those in love. In the context of the romance, John seizes the opportunity to enjoy aspects of himself that he has rarely experienced. Unrecognized self-discovery is a sizable component in the thrill of any romance. Being American, however, he assumes that it is the girl who thrills him.

Among the activities traditionally reserved for romance is the exploration of sexual capacity. Whether the couple copulate or not, there is a sexual focus in romance. John is not a complete novice to sex, but he expects to find it more rewarding with someone he loves; moreover, Mary corresponds to his particularized conception of a desirable sexual partner.

Like most Americans, John also sexualizes his desire to repossess the alienated qualities which he has projected onto his beloved. The lover wants to make these characteristics a part of himself, to reunite with his alienated potential. But, because he thinks of these things as aspects of his sweetheart, he assumes that his desire is to unite with her—a phrase which in America is a euphemism for sexual relations. Following his culture's definitions and interpretations, John develops a *sexualized* interest in Mary which is quite independent of his biological urgings.

John has projected so much of himself onto Mary that he is miserable without her. He is jealous of anyone else who is close to her, for he wants exclusive and constant possession of the potential he projects onto her.

Mary is in a similar state. She finds and loves in John many qualities which she has alienated from her self-image: poise, wit, forcefulness, self-assurance. She, too, has an Ideal, composed of conventional as well as idiosyncratic projections, of many things she would like to be but is sure she is not. She hangs this image on John and finds that he is wonderful.

Moreover, finding someone who thinks that *she* is wonderful is a balm to ease her self-doubts. As an adjusted American girl, Mary has learned to seek self-acceptance indirectly, through winning approval, admiration, and love from others. John's love for her seems the epitome of acceptance, and Mary clings to it.

Because each wants to be loved, each agrees to love the other (not that the bargain is explicit, of course, but it is understood all the same). Like most lovers, these two form a mutual admiration society, dedicated to indirect self-acceptance. No romance is ever open and candid, for both parties are intent on making and maintaining a good impression. Mary seems a fault-less angel to John because he is seeing what he has projected onto her—a view she encourages by seeking to conceal less flattering characteristics and by trying to fit his picture of her. Anything he praises, she seeks to emphasize, and because he compliments her on what he expects to see (independently of reality) she finds herself cultivating new and exciting self-poten-tial.

All of this could lead to self-discovery on Mary's part. As realists have long noted, the appearance and disposition of an unattractive shrewish girl can be re-markably improved by daily assertions that she is beautiful and sweet tempered. Mary would like to believe the image of herself that she sees reflected in John's eyes. But she knows that she is concealing other facets of herself (perhaps ill-tempered or slov-enly proclivities) and, moreover, she finds it hard to believe that the charms John attributes to her are real. Any changes which she does perceive in herself she believes are elicited by John, and she fears that if she lost him she *might* turn into a pumpkin. So she clings to him as a prop for a masquerade she hopes will never end. Her self-discovery remains unrecog-nized.

Mary has yet another reason for wanting to believe that she is in love. Having learned a contradictory set of ideas about sex, she is ambivalent about the sexual nature of the romance. She is uneasy about being sexually aroused and thinks that, if her feeling for John is only infatuation, her awakening sexual inter-ests are dangerous and wrong. But she believes that if her feeling is Love she ought to desire him. Since she does find herself desiring him, she feels she had bet-ter be in love, and any questions about the suitability of marriage with John are pushed out of her mind.

John and Mary are in love, and they believe it is neither possible nor desirable to know why. But, as adjusted Americans, they are confident that love and marriage go together, and so they are wed.

The Marriage of John and Mary

Although evidence is abundant, it is seldom remarked that the degree to which people are in love when they marry is not correlated to the amount of pleasure they derive from marriage. Some who were wildly in love find disappointment, and some who were never in love find happiness—but the reverse can also be true. The fact is that marital bliss depends on other variables than love, although love may complicate marital adjustment.

John and Mary have been married several years. The excitement of engagement and marriage rituals and the thrill of setting up housekeeping are forgotten, and both of them would admit that the honeymoon is over. More precisely, the nature of their relationship has changed. Self-discovery has atrophied, largely because they no longer exercise initiative in enjoying themselves as they did during their romance. The unflattering light of continual association makes it difficult for either to maintain an idealized image of the other, and each is well aware that the other no longer thinks he is perfect.

Moreover, they have begun to hang negative projections on each other. Unlike a True Love, a spouse is a convenient depository for undesired aspects of the self. For example, John feels trapped by mounting expenses. His own desire to spend recklessly seems threatening, so he projects it onto Mary and finds her demanding and extravagant.

Mary is still caught up in her ambivalence about sex. She projects onto her husband her desire to experiment sexually, then complains that he is intent on pressuring her into sexual variations. This is a traditional middle-class pattern, and it is probable that her mother and her grandmother made similar projections and complaints.

But, because Mary is a modern wife, her sex life is complicated further by her belief (acquired from marriage manuals) that her adequacy as a woman is measured by her sexual competence and the degree to which she enjoys intercourse. Her natural desire to enjoy sex is obscured by the feeling that she *ought* to enjoy it. She alternates between avoiding sexual relations and concentrating so intently on achieving orgasm that there is little pleasure in the process.

In these sexual complications, John is no help. The same marriage manuals have informed him that he has a choice between being a selfish, brutal male, and being a sympathetic, competent lover who makes sure that he gives full satisfaction to his partner. Wanting to be a sympathetic, competent lover, he becomes hyperconscious of her response. He watches her to see how much pleasure he is able to give her, and Mary watches him watching her. Proving his competence by giving her pleasure becomes so important to him that his own enjoyment is greatly reduced. Moreover, his preoccupation with her response encourages her idea that sexual excitement is something she ought to feel in order not to disappoint John. (She sometimes finds herself thinking that life and sex might be simpler if her husband were a selfish, brutal male who allowed her to respond or not as she pleased.)

Finally, as their positive projections on each other have dimmed, so has the sexualized desire to repossess them. With sexualization gone, they are left with only the sexual urge itself, a fact which they manage to regard as a sign of sexual incompatibility.

Yet, during this same period, they are achieving a general adaptation to each other, a growing acceptance of each other's quirks, even (in spite of their confusions) some sexual competence. They no longer feel the need for pretense with each other, or at least they have largely abandoned efforts to maintain it. The way is opening for a candid intimacy. Moreover, they are building ties of mutual need satisfaction. Any advance either of them could make in understanding himself and his needs would be richly rewarded in their enjoyment of each other.

But John and Mary are more aware of the dissolution of old ties based on love than of the emergence of new ones founded on mutual need satisfaction. Mary feels threatened by the changing nature of her relation to her husband and (projecting her doubts onto him) asks at odd moments, "Do you still love me?" John has his own doubts about his feelings, and the question serves to magnify them. Preoccupied with what they believe are interpersonal failures, they do not perceive the intrapersonal origin of their difficulties.

The specific quarrels that John and Mary have are largely irrelevant; even if by fortuitous amnesia they were able to forget and begin their marriage anew, their love would not last. The simple fact is that the adulterous aristocrats of the Middle Ages were right: marriage is corrosive to love.

And love is an impediment to marital happiness. Founded on projection, abetting the quest for indirect self-acceptance, love can contribute neither to candid intimacy nor to self-acceptance. But, like most of their adjusted compatriots, this couple believe that love is the only basis for marriage. As they feel love evaporating, they begin to wonder if their marriage was a mistake. In their concern for love, they blind themselves to the possible success of their marriage.

The True Love of John and Sue

It has become apparent that John's Ideal image was not a good fit on Mary (he would say that Mary has changed) and, without letting himself recognize what he is doing, he has been looking for someone else on whom he can project it. Sue happens to be handy, and although familiarity may erode love, propinquity helps initiate it. So the time comes when John transfers to Sue the sides of himself which he once had projected onto Mary. He interprets the transfer as the discovery that Sue is his Ideal, and he feels drawn to her.

John wants to repossess alienated sides of himself which he has not enjoyed even vicariously since his troubles with his wife began. As before, he interprets this feeling as a desire to possess the girl on whom he projects the beloved but alienated sides of himself— and thus he sexualizes the attraction. John's sexual needs are easily and conveniently satisfied with his spouse (or at least could be if he would quit worrying about being a sympathetic, competent lover). But, having projected onto Sue qualities that he wants to make part of himself he thinks he wants to "make" Sue.

This desire is disturbing to John, for part of his self-image involves being an ethical man. During his marriage he has experienced fleeting desires for other women, but nothing like the intense desire produced by the sexualization of his projections on Sue. Not comprehending the nature of his attraction, he has trouble reconciling it with his desire to be a faithful husband. The myth of love resolves his dilemma with a comforting rationalization: having learned to regard love as unpredictable, irresistible, and involuntary, he can argue that if he is in love with the girl he is noble for hiding his feelings, rather than guilty for having them. Quite predictably, he falls in love with Sue.

This is the mechanism of the Great Romance. The married individual projects desired potential onto someone other than his spouse, is drawn to it, sexualizes the attraction, then rationalizes the resulting adulterous desire by claiming it to be the flowering of True Love. This is the Great Romance of his life, and how can he deny himself and his beloved? This pattern is common among adjusted Americans, and John falls into it and into his first affair.

In his romance with Sue, he recaptures many of the pleasures he had once known with Mary. He experiences again the flattering role of the lover, to which tabu adds relish. And he enjoys the positive projections that Sue hangs on him. Even if he discounts her view of him, it is a joy to find again someone who thinks he is wonderful. Gratefully, he reciprocates.

But in spite of the excitement of his new romance, John is confused and unhappy. He feels that he has a right to his Great Romance, and he feels that he is a heel. His thoughts of how unfair his unfaithfulness is to Mary are countered by thoughts of how unfair it is to remain with her when he and Sue really love each other. In the end, he runs from the conflict by projecting onto his wife his own desire to remain with her, and experiencing it as if it were possessiveness on her part. He becomes convinced that all *he* wants to do is to divorce Mary and marry Sue. He laments the fact that he did not meet Sue first—never dreaming that, if he had, the partner in his Great Romance might well have been Mary.

The True Love of Mary and Bill

As Mary first suspects and then discovers her husband's extramarital adventure, she finds in it proof of her own inadequacy. Her self-doubts seem confirmed, and her need to find herself acceptable mounts. She becomes increasingly tense, a feeling which she interprets as anger. Following the line of cultural expectation, she turns her tension into tearful denunciation of her unfaithful spouse.

Were Mary capable of direct self-acceptance, the situation might develop quite differently. It might still be difficult for Mary to avoid some emotional entanglement in John's confusion, but if she were self-accepting she could ease him over his Great Romance. With time, John would discover that his projections fit Sue no better than Mary. He is accustomed to satisfying many needs with his wife, and in the long run would probably recognize that the ties to Mary are stronger than the attraction to Sue.

But feeling threatened and wronged, Mary pulls away from her husband. She refuses to satisfy needs with John as a means of punishing him, and the result is that she deprives herself and becomes more needful, tense, and angry. At the same time, she is breaking the ties of mutual need satisfaction that could have held John.

Many an indignant wife has consulted a lawyer at this point, but Mary is as anxious to ease her feelings of inadequacy as she is to punish John. In some societies the children she has borne would be proof of her adequacy as a woman, but Mary is an American and believes that the proof of her femininity is her ability to appeal and to respond to men sexually. After several years of washing diapers, scrubbing sinks, and scolding children, Mary feels more like a bedraggled housemaid than an enticing female.

In an effort to prove to herself that she can still be attractive, Mary splurges on a startling dress and a new hair style, and goes to a party alone (John had declined the invitation, pleading that he had to work late). It is not surprising that men should begin paying Mary compliments, although she would not want to admit that she had invited their advances. An acquaintance named Bill soon monopolizes her, and for the moment, at least, her self-doubts are eased. She slips out of the party with Bill and sets out to do the town. She has not experienced the "orchids and champagne" Mary in years, but she expects to recapture this feeling with Bill—and so she does.

Part of her self-image involves being a faithful wife in spite of what John may do, and she has never thought that she would become involved in an affair. Like John, she is ambivalent. But she alienates her disapproval, and her scruples then seem an unreasonable demand by "society" that she be faithful when her husband is not. Bill assures her that the double standard went out with bloomers and Mary is ready to agree.

In the abandon of an affair, Mary ceases to regard sex as something she *ought* to enjoy and begins to think of it as something she *wants* to enjoy. The result is that she makes some startling discoveries about her own capacity for sexual enjoyment. However, she fails to perceive that her enjoyment is the result of her own attitude and behavior, and assumes that it is a consequence of having changed partners. It distresses her to feel guilty about her new-found pleasure in sex. She is soon able to rationalize it by discovering that her affair with Bill is the Great Romance of *her* life.

The rebellious affair helps Mary to experiment sexually, but it inhibits any self-understanding. Even during periods when she thinks she would like to make her marriage work, she finds it difficult to admit that her Great Romance could be motivated by hostile retaliation. Besides, the positive projections she now hangs on Bill convince her that she really loves him. Before long, Mary is too far out on the limb of loving Bill to get back.

John is jealous, but at the same time he finds his wife's affair a convenient justification for his own behavior. He can assure himself that he and Mary were incompatible after all, and that both of them will surely be happier married to their new loves. So the marriage of John and Mary ends, but (barring unlikely insight) their future may be more predictable than either of them realizes.

On whom will John hang his idealized projections after he becomes disillusioned with Sue? Recoiling from a second divorce, he may settle down in resignation. Or he may pursue his idealized projections and marry again and again. But the person agonizing over the decision of divorcing his spouse to marry his love is likely to miss the crux of the problem, which is the unsuitability of love as a foundation for marriage. Those who long to stay in love forever seldom stay married for long.

Beyond Love

Some people would object that the concept of love we have employed is too narrow, that love is more than this. Certainly the attraction between two people may involve any one or a combination of different mechanisms: mutual admiration, reciprocal rationalization, unrecognized self-discovery, localized self-acceptance, or mutual need satisfaction, as well as the projection of alienated but desired characteristics. It would be possible to define love as involving some combination of these, or to designate the forms of attraction as $love_1$, $love_2$, $love_3$, etc. This would not alter the analysis, only the terminology.

For the sake of clarity, we have restricted the word *love* to that attraction which is based on the projection of alienated but desired characteristics. Such projection leads to an intense desire to be with the person on whom the projections are hung, to exhilaration when he is present, to depression when he is absent, to possesive jealousy. Our usage is thus consistent with the kind of feeling an American usually has in mind when he says, "I love you."

Love thus defined is a major factor in the American's choice of spouse, but if those who marry for love find happiness, it is more in spite of love than because of it. Without comprehending what they are doing, they must overcome the projections of love which lead away from self-knowledge and blur their perceptions of each other. They must make a transition from this to the candor and understanding of at least a localized self-acceptance.

But most couples assume that happiness will come to them if only they marry the one they love, and thus they are more concerned with clinging to love than with building a rewarding marriage. The assumption that the spouse is the source of pleasure in marriage leads the individual to blame his spouse when he fails to find the pleasure he had expected. As long as he makes this assumption, he is likely to look for another spouse instead of altering the behaviors through which he seeks marital satisfaction.

The parties to a successful marriage learn *to expect to enjoy the self in marriage rather than to expect to enjoy the spouse*. Because the expectation is different, the interaction is different. As each partner seeks to maximize his own enjoyment of the marriage, he assists his spouse in doing the same. Each is seeking candor and warmth, and the exploration of self-potential (sexual capacities and many others), all of which is facilitated by the cooperation of someone else engaged in a similar development. Such persons are not preoccupied with being loved or with maintaining romantic illusions. They are trying to enjoy life—together.

It may be that the phrase "mature love" is sometimes intended to convey the idea of this kind of relationship, but if so the usage is misleading, for it implies that the so-called "mature love" is a natural outgrowth of romantic love. This is hardly the case, for love leads in the opposite direction. It is no accident that the greatest tales of love end with the death of the lovers; there is simply no other plausible ending that would not conflict with the myth of love. Love may form the basis for a charming weekend, but it is an unstable foundation for a marriage.

The American has difficulty imagining how he would choose a mate apart from the compulsion of love. Actually, the specific person he marries is less important to his happiness than he believes—the attitudes with which he approaches marriage are far more significant. The person who sees marriage as an opportunity for experiencing the warm, demonstrative potential in himself, and for satisfying needs in a candid and stable association, usually finds what he seeks. The general rule is that people who enjoy life enjoy marriage. Some people would be unhappy with any spouse, for they do not allow themselves happiness. A few other people would be happy almost regardless of whom they married. The large middle group, however, is most likely to find marital happiness if they seek a spouse who has an unusual degree of self-understanding and self-acceptance.

The idea of moving beyond love is initially frightening to most Americans, once they grasp that love itself is being challenged, and not just romantic illusion. Many people fear that analysis of their loves would undermine the sense of being loved that seems so essential in their pursuit of indirect self-acceptance. Others regret the effect of insight on the poetic aura which surrounds love. Yet love is at best a temporary euphoria, and the individual who pursues it finds it impossible to seize and hold. The quest for love, like the quest for indirect self-acceptance, is a neurotic pattern—an impediment to the fulfillment it falsely promises.

II
THE PROBLEM OF
PARENTAL LOVE

*Thou art young, and desirest child and marriage. But
I ask thee:
Art thou a man entitled to desire a child?
Art thou the victorious one, the self-conqueror, the
ruler of thy passions, the master of thy virtues? Thus
do I ask thee.
Or doth the animal speak in thy wish, and necessity?
Or isolation? Or discord in thee?* FRIEDRICH NIETZSCHE

*. . . out of some forty families I have been able to
observe, I know hardly four in which the parents do
not act in such a way that nothing would be more desirable for the child than to escape their influence.*

ANDRÉ GIDE

A certain amount of love for one's young is probably
inevitable, but there is little profit for either parent
or child in encouraging or glorifying it. That such a
statement may seem irresponsible, if not downright
immoral, indicates the degree to which love has become a sacred cow in American culture. Most Americans are only too aware that their interaction with
their children is not what they might wish, but they
fail to perceive the source and meaning of most of

their difficulties. Uncritical adulation of parental love blinds them.

Love is probably the emotion most talked about and extolled by Americans and probably also the least understood. In large measure this is because love seems a natural human emotion that requires no explanation. It is taken for granted that love for one's spouse and children is a univeral element in human experience, something that men of all places and ages have felt in common. Affection and warmth are universal, to be sure, but not love in the middle-class sense of the word. What seems to be a natural emotional response is largely a conventional response.

The range of human emotional potential is broad, and that set of responses which is accorded the highest value in one society may not be highly regarded in another. Thus, filial piety was considered the finest emotion in traditional Chinese society, patriotism was the transcendent emotion in ancient Sparta, the Puritans extolled the fear of God above all else, and the modern Americans exalt love.

As it would have seemed sacrilege to the Puritan to suggest that man approach God in any attitude but fear, so it seems sacrilege to the modern American to suggest that the parent approach his child with anything but love. In America, love is regarded not only as man's finest feeling but also as a prime mover. The American tends to assume that whatever is not done for money is surely done for love, and when he says that he would not do something "for love or money" he means that he would not do it at all.

Americans differentiate many levels and types of love, for much the same reason that the Arabian nomads had a thousand words for "sword." But the underlying psychological mechanism of love is essentially the same whether the love in question be called puppy love, mature love, romantic love, platonic love, parental love, or any other relationship that involves adoration of one person by another.

What happens, in essence, is that one person projects some part of himself which he values highly onto someone else, where he adores it. He then begins to act as if this person were an extension of himself. Longing to enjoy the misplaced part of himself, he clings to the person on whom he has projected it, he is possessive and jealous, he delights in the loved one's presence, but feels anxious and incomplete when this person is absent. Stated thus baldly, love may sound neither very admirable nor enjoyable. But this is nevertheless the kind of feeling the American has in mind when he says, "I love you."

There are many parallels between romantic love, the subject of the last chapter, and parental love. In the same way that the American learns to consider certain attributes appropriate and desirable for one sex but unacceptable for the other, so he learns to consider certain qualities endearing in children but inappropriate for adults. Children can be affectionate, warm, and dependent in ways that most adults do not permit themselves to be. Children can feel free to do outrageous things such as rolling in the mud or being rude to visiting relatives. And children can loaf and play, free from responsibility.

The capacity and the desire to behave like a child are not lost by the adult; they are supplemented by, and ultimately subordinated to, the adult self image, but they remain as latent potential. Often the adult has a rigid and narrow conception of maturity that excludes his childlike potential. Yet the proper adult has his impish side still, and refusing to recognize it does not obliterate it. The adult who has sexualized and alienated his desire to cuddle and be cuddled may be stiffly aloof most of the time, but his desire remains. And the adult who bristles with independence has merely alienated a strong desire to be dependent on others. These and other alienated characteristics are customarily projected onto children, in whom such desires and behaviors are deemed appropriate.

Some adults are so concerned with holding their childlike potential at a distance that they are uncomfortable with the children on whom they project it. These are the adults who confess that they simply do not enjoy children. But most adults find their childlike potential amusing, charming, and *lovable* when projected onto children—particularly when the children involved are their own. The desire to experience vicariously and to indulge projected childlike facets of the self is one of the basic ingredients of parental love.

The desire to re-create the self through one's child is another important factor in parental love. Recoiling from the thought of his own death, the parent seeks to cheat the grave by creating himself anew in his offspring. While he is about it, he hopes to make some improvements. He hangs on the child his own unrealized potential and sees not the child but the projected image of the person he would like to be. The loving parent has clothed his child with a great deal of himself, and he clings to the child possessively.

Often, as in romantic love, the desire to repossess projected aspects of the self is interpreted as a desire to unite physically with the person on whom they are projected. Such a desire is usually given a sexual interpretation. However, incestuous desire is highly tabu in American culture, as is sexual interest in children. The effect of these tabus is to drive from consciousness the sexualization of love for the child. It is then experienced via projection, and the parent may become preoccupied with curbing what seems to him the child's precocious sexual interests, or with protecting his child from sexual interests he attributes to the child's playmates or to sex perverts. (This is not to deny that the latter two groups—or the child himself—have sexual interests. It is rather to note that they are often targets for the projected sexual interests which the parent is unwilling to admit are his own.)

The American father is generally more inhibited in fondling his children than is the mother. He is also more prone to assuming that his interest in physical contact with them is sexual in nature. He is likely to practice a studied avoidance of physical contact with any child past puberty, the age at which (in American mythology) the child is transformed from a sexless creature to a sexual one. And in the case of a male child, the father's fear of homosexuality is added to the fear of incestuous desire. He is terrified at the thought of being physically attracted to a young boy and is likely to be awkward and inhibited in any physical contact he has with his son. Thus, parental love (that is, the parent's emotional involvement with qualities he has projected onto his child) is likely to have suppressed sexual undertones. This means that love can actually inhibit the expression of physical warmth between parent and child, particularly between a father and his adolescent son.

Love is essentially a neurotic response. A neurosis is an internal, nonorganic barrier to need fulfillment, and love arises in the parent because of his incapacity to satisfy his need for an accurate and acceptable self-image. When he has induced comparable problems in his child, the child will reciprocate this love.

The adjusted American experiences tension and conflict in parenthood and is concerned about it. If his home contains few books, it will still be likely to have a cross-indexed volume on how to raise children. Yet the underlying source of much of the conflict escapes recognition because it is a normal neurosis. Holding love to be of all emotions the most elevated, the American blinds himself to the deleterious effects that love has on his relations with his family—indeed, he struggles to overcome these effects by loving them more.

What Does the Lamb Say?

There is the common case of the devoted mother who is preoccupied with a small daughter whom she deeply loves. The mother lives a restricted life. Taking the toddler anywhere is an exhausting experience for both, and when visitors come the child manages to preempt most of her mother's attention. As this mother sees it, the needs of her baby leave little time for doing things with other people, or for herself. She recognizes that not all women are so monopolized by their children, but views this as evidence that other mothers are less conscientious than she. She insists that a child needs its mother's full attention and that she loves her baby so much she is glad to devote her life to her child. The latter is true enough.

Chronically uncertain about her capacity to succeed at anything, this woman worried during pregnancy about whether she could be a good mother. From the time she came home from the hospital (apprehensive about being on her own with the baby), she has been preoccupied with trying to prove that she is an adequate parent. Motherhood has come to dominate her self-image—significantly, she usually refers to herself as "Mommy."

Devoting herself to her baby, this mother begins to identify with the child and to hang all manner of projections on her. She is convinced that her daughter will be pretty and talented (she has always thought of herself as plain and inept). She resolves to make certain that her daughter develops her potential. Having projected so much of herself onto her daughter, she finds the child's presence indispensable—but she is not clinging to the child, only to her projections. She wants to be with her daughter continuously to enjoy vicariously, to encourage, and to protect the alienated facets of herself with which she has endowed her daughter.

There is another element in the relationship, also deriving from the mother's self-doubts. By spending most of her time talking baby talk and playing with her baby, this woman is able to escape from adult interaction. She retreats into a pseudo-childhood, with the comforting rationalization that her actions are those of a loving mother. In the process her doubts about her capacity to function as an adult are aggravated. The little girl, meanwhile, is prevented from experimenting with her own childhood.

In spite of this mother's devotion, the child's needs are often left unsatisfied. They are ignored by the mother, who insists that the child satisfy needs which the mother projects onto her. Picture the mother, the child, and the father as they go for a drive in the country. The mother is delighted to get out (hers is a confining life) but from the time the car rolls down the driveway she devotes herself to "making the ride fun for the baby." Her own desires to see and to enjoy are projected onto the child, whom she holds up to the window.

Before long the little girl begins to squirm and says "night-night," her signal that she is sleepy. The mother ignores the request (*she* is not tired) and burbles, "See the cow? Isn't that a pretty cow?" The child is not looking. With still greater animation the fond parent tries to rekindle interest. "See the little lamb! What does the lamb say?"

"Go night-night!"

Only when the exhausted baby is tense and fussing does the mother decide to put her on the back seat for a nap. By this time, however, the child is no longer relaxed enough to sleep. The mother struggles to quiet her, but a howling baby, a frantic mother, and a profane father return from the ride.

Boys Will Be Boys

Parental love also interferes with the child's struggle to grow up. Here is the mother who worries about having sent her only son to camp. She is certain that he will lose his clothes, forget to brush his teeth, be neglected by the counselors, and become homesick. For the sake of argument, let us grant that her predictions are essentially correct. But if her son is less able to take care of himself than other boys are, it is because he has never had a chance to learn. He is accustomed to his mother's loving care.

The key to this mother's love is the projection of her own irresponsible, dependent qualities onto her son. In accordance with major aspects of her self-image, she takes pride in being a responsible, orderly, and self-sacrificing adult. But an alienated part of her would like to be demanding and selfish, to strew things about, and to let others worry about the consequences of her actions.

This woman was raised to believe that children—particularly boys—have a right to be and to do such things, and she projects her alienated desire to be dependent and undisciplined onto her son. When she indulges him she is indulging the aspects of herself which she has hung on him. In effect, she encourages him to be irresponsible and demanding, and, in time, her projections are a good fit. When her husband complains about the boy's behavior she defends the child, contending that his actions "only prove that he is all boy."

Because she cherishes the childlike facets of herself which she experiences through her son, and because she allows herself no other or more direct enjoyment of these aspects of herself, she has no wish to see him grow up. When her husband declares that it is time the boy learned to assume responsibility, she answers, "Children grow up too soon, why crowd him?" She loves her son as she has created him—demanding, irresponsible, and careless.

Typically, the more a child is loved the less he is enjoyed. The loved child has little chance to learn to amuse himself or to develop independence. He learns only to expect the continuous attention of his loving parent, and he becomes a demanding child. His demands, when added to those that the parent projects onto him, amount to a staggering total. However much the parent may welcome an opportunity to indulge his projected childlike nature, there is another side to his feelings: resentment.

Yet this emotion is unacceptable to the loving parent, and he (or she) recoils from it. Commonly, such a parent denies that the resentment exists, while simultaneously becoming a doormat for the child as a means of atoning for it. The wear and tear endured while serving as a doormat increase the resentment, and a vicious circle is set spinning.

The parent is likely to try to conceal his resentment from himself by projecting it. The mother who encourages her child to be demanding and careless is likely to be certain that all those who have contact with her son are annoyed by his demands and his carelessness. Such projections may fit, but it is nevertheless her own resentment against which she sputters and fumes—and from which she attempts to shield the boy. If her husband openly resents the child, she will have a convenient place to hang her own resentment, and the child will become a focal point for marital conflict.

Some Go Wrong

The American parent expects his child to be a source of emotional satisfaction and hopes to find his relationship to his child a deeply meaningful experience. He assumes that such hopes and expectations are natural, and if he finds that he does not love his child he is disturbed. The resentment a new father feels when his wife is suddenly monopolized by an infant and the guilt the new father feels about his resentment are familiar. But we are here concerned with a more complex pattern, in which a father who was once devoted to his small son comes to reject the boy as he grows older and to be concerned about his inability to love him.

Frequently such a father is seeking immortality and vicarious fulfillment of his own undeveloped capacities through his son. It is easy to see almost any potential in a tiny child, and a father's projections on his infant son can take any direction he fancies. Thus, the father may be tremendously attached to his small son. But inevitably as the boy grows older he develops a self of his own—and not precisely the self that his father had in mind. The father demands that the son succeed where he himself has failed and develop qualities which the father has allowed to remain latent. When the son does not, the father is disappointed.

When it becomes abundantly clear that projections do not fit the person on whom they are hung, love cools abruptly. The husband who finds that his wife does not fit his image of the ideal woman (a composite image of cherished qualities he has alienated from himself) may begin to look ardently at women who are unfamiliar enough to seem to fit his projections. Similarly, the father who perceives that his fond hopes are not being realized in his son may begin to make invidious comparisons between his son and other boys who are distant enough to seem sterling lads.

Because the father believes that he *should* love his son, he is disturbed when he finds that he does not. He feels that there must be either something wrong with himself or something unlovable about the boy. The latter is the more palatable possibility to the father, and so he finds fault with his son. He can always find shortcomings in the boy to explain why the latter is unlovable. For one, there is the fact that the boy is turning out poorly (that is, he is no improvement on his father).

He is likely to find his son demanding and ungrateful. He tries to give his son opportunities that he himself did not have as a child (wanting to participate vicariously in an idealized childhood). But losing sight of his motivation, he assumes that these are things he does for the boy and he expects gratitude. Because things the father would like if he were a child again do not necessarily appeal to his son, the boy is not always grateful for his "advantages." The father points out that his son takes things for granted (being accustomed to having them showered upon him), does not appreciate things (not having particularly wanted them), or asks for something more (having his own ideas of what he wants in *his* childhood).

The conflicts between this father and son are in large measure a result of the father's attempts to love his child and to rationalize his failure to do so. The father alternates between trying to make his son fit the image he is prepared to love and, failing in this, trying to prove that the boy is simply not lovable.

The Little Tin God

The expectation that the child will love the parent is one of the covert motives which lead the adjusted American to want children. Insecure and longing for approval, the parent hopes that he can raise someone to love and admire him. The ancient commandment "Honor thy father and thy mother" has been subtly altered in American culture to "Love thy father and thy mother."

The child is aware of his dependence on his parent for physical and emotional sustenance, and, perceiving his parent as the bringer of satisfactions and the righter of wrongs, he values him. But he also perceives the parent as the imposer of restrictions and punishments, and he fears and resents him. The inherent nature of the relationship between parent and child leads to ambivalent emotions. However, the American child soon learns that he is expected to conceal his fear and anger responses and to reciprocate his parent's love.

There is an element of love in the child's feeling for the parent, and it is similar to all other forms of love. The child finds in his parent qualities which he believes are not in himself and which he longs to make a part of himself. Insofar as this results in the child taking the parent as a model, this is a functional emotion. If the child is given assurance that in time he can develop capacities similar to those he admires in his father (or mother), hero worship of the parent can contribute to the child's development of a viable self-image. *But this development requires that the child become aware of his own latent potential.*

The parent who seeks indirect self-acceptance

through the child's love is more likely to encourage the hero worship for its own sake than to turn it toward the child's development. This may be the only hero worship he has even received, and he may unconsciously exploit it.

Such a parent is likely to overwhelm his child, playing off the child's puny efforts against his own, engaging in games with him (in the name of being a "pal" to his son) but excelling without teaching. By continuously displaying his skill in comparison to the child's he squeezes the last drop of adoration from him but at the expense of the child's self-confidence.

When the parent plays God in a small universe, he expects his child to worship him. But a child who seems to do so actually worships his own unrecognized potential. Projecting his own latent strength and skills onto his parent, he sees himself as weak and bungling. He then cries out for the parent to accept him, for he cannot accept himself.

Yet the parent who creates such a needful child is singularly unlikely to grant the approval his child seeks. The child tries desperately to be "perfect," for he thinks that perfection would bring the coveted acceptance from the parent. But small steps in the learning process are all that he is likely to achieve in a short space of time, and these small improvements are likely to elicit from such a parent only impatient remarks about how slowly the child is progressing. (After all, this parent would feel threatened by any real success on the part of the child.) Long before the child has approached even a small measure of perfection, he is likely to quit in tearful shame. Pinning his hopes for acceptance on intense but spasmodic efforts to acquire some skill, then retreating in shame and self-doubt may become a pattern for the child. Repeated in various areas of activity, the pattern leads to an overwhelming sense of failure and personal inadequacy. The future course of the child's life is sadly predictable.

A variant of this kind of parent worship occurs when one parent holds the other up as a model. An occasional mother may hold up her husband to her son as the epitome of all that is manly, hiding his imperfections. She may feel that the father has too little contact with the son for the latter to be able to see his father's best qualities, and so she makes a point of qualities which she would like to see the boy emulate. (These are likely to be qualities which she has projected onto her husband.) But whatever the mother's motives, the effect is pernicious. The son will either try to protect his tenuous self-acceptance by refusing to accept his father as a model, or will lose sight of his own potential and worship his father from a vast psychological distance.

Because the parent is inevitably stronger and more skillful than the small child, such a parent-worshiping relationship may continue its neurotic course for a number of years. The child may never feel capable of achieving the same level of skill as his father and may languish in the parental shadow all his life. The sons of famous fathers are often caught up in this pattern. Their family (and outsiders) may expect them to repeat their father's achievements, but a lifelong sense of being inferior to the father may leave such sons incapable of developing their own potential.

More frequently, the time comes when the adolescent boy begins to feel that his childhood image of his father was false, or at least inflated. The father appears as a fraud and the son feels cheated. But although the boy may experience a sense of loss when he becomes aware that his view of his father has been exaggerated, he does not necessarily acquire thereby an awareness of his own latent capacities. He may simply come to feel that his father, too, is a bungling incompetent.

The child who sees his parent less as a hero and more as a human being can take his parent as a model. As a small child he is less likely to adore his father, but as an adolescent he is less likely to scorn him. And he is very likely to become aware of his own potential at an early age.

The Child beyond Love

Undeniably, the human infant needs more than food, drink, and sanitation. A child seems to require a considerable amount of physical handling and comforting. Simply being in bodily contact with its mother seems to be important to the small child. In cultures where infants are carried most of the time next to their mothers' bodies it is rare to hear a baby cry. Experiments on human babies are generally frowned upon, but monkey babies have been raised in experimental situations with a surrogate mother made of wire and terry cloth (and a feeding bottle). These monkeys show extreme anxiety when deprived of physical contact with their "mother." Clinging to the source of physical satisfaction seems to characterize small primates.

This is presumably the need long since noted by the advocates of "tender, loving care." But the infant's need is more for tender, frequent handling than for the kind of emotional involvement most American parents have in mind when they talk about loving their children. For all their concern about their children, Americans exercise an amazing restraint on bodily contact with them. In striking contrast is the relation between parents and children in many "underdeveloped" cultures. In a survey conducted in a rural region of Mexico, people were asked to indicate their favorite and most frequent pastimes. Far and away the most frequent answer to both questions was "playing with my children." And this did not mean organizing ball games or hand-craft activities; this meant tossing and tussling and physical fondling.

Too often, the American parent communicates to his child at a tender age the idea that he should not press himself on others too demonstratively, and the child turns his impulse to touch and fondle others into more aggressive contact. The tabu on fondling is reinforced shortly by the kindergarten teacher who bears down on the matter of "keeping your hands to yourself." The final product is an individual who is almost incapable of expressing warmth physically. Thus one inhibited generation inhibits the next.

And thus the American parent is likely to find it difficult to give his children the fondling they need simply because he (or she) has never learned to express physical warmth. Moreover, the love relationship itself may inhibit warm physical contact between parent and child, for it is likely to aggravate the parent's buried fears that his desire to handle the child may have a sexual basis.

The child's love for the parent and the parent's love for the child are generally stultifying to the child and disappointing to the parent. Moreover, love is ever one side of a basic ambivalence. To love one's child is also to resent him. Yet, being creatures of their culture, adjusted Americans assume that the only alternatives to loving a child are rejection and indifference. Happily this is not the case. Indeed, rejection and indifference most often derive from an unsatisfying attempt at loving a child.

Interest in children can be founded in love (although the parent who loves his child may scarcely know what the child under the projections is like). But interest in a child can also be founded in a healthy self-interest. Being a good parent is an important part of the self-image of most adults, and children provide the opportunity to explore and enjoy his potentiality of the self.

This motivation can lead the parent to a variety of behaviors, some constructive, some destructive. If he insists that his child achieve and behave so that he, the parent, will appear to be a splendid parent in the eyes of the community, the result will be continuous and destructive interference with the life of the child. But the same motivation can lead to a richly rewarding relation between parent and child if the former conceives being a good parent as a matter of helping the child discover his capacities and develop a viable self-image. Seeking to develop his own capacity for being an effective parent, he will discover that shaping a child can be fascinating. As the sculptor draws out and enhances the beauty inherent in his medium, so the parent can elicit and encourage the inherent qualities of his child. Leading a child to self-discovery is a creative art. It is also a delightful activity.

The parent who has learned to live his own life fully makes an incalculable contribution to the development of his child. Because the child imitates his parents' neurotic and healthful patterns alike, it is a fortunate child who has the opportunity to take as a model a parent who effectively satisfies his own needs. Moreover, the parent who has achieved insight into his own neuroses will be able to give dignity to his child's problems.

The relationship between parent and child will inevitably have tempestuous moments, if only because of the controls which the parent must impose for the child's safety. But on balance the relationship can be warm, accepting, and rewarding for all concerned, if the complexities of love are not added. The parent who does not love/resent his child can establish a pattern of mutual need satisfaction with him. In his parental role he finds self-acceptance through acting on capacities he values; the child in turn discovers and accepts himself through interaction with his parent. Such relationships are rare between American parents and children but not uncommon between a boy and his favorite uncle.

It must be underscored that interaction based on mutually rewarding behaviors is *not* an exalted stage of parental love. It is founded on an entirely different basis: on habits of mutual need satisfaction and self-acceptance. Such a relationship is not love and lacks love's detrimental effects.

12
THE WEIGHT OF OBLIGATION

If you begin by sacrificing yourself to those you love, you will end by hating those to whom you have sacrificed yourself. GEORGE BERNARD SHAW

Electra: "I'm not marrying anyone, I've got my duty to Father." EUGENE O'NEILL

Americans often feel that their freedom of choice is largely hypothetical, that obligations to others (children, parents, creditors, and the like) prevent them from exercising it. Some assume obligations dutifully, some resentfully, but nearly all would tend to agree on two points: that men must be bound by obligations if society is to function, and that these obligations impose self-sacrifice on the individual. Both assumptions are questionable.

Men would probably take better care of each other if the idea of obligation were quietly laid aside, and self-sacrifice is not what it appears to be. The "self-sacrificing" person is motivated by his own desires, not by devotion to duty or by the needs of others. He who is preoccupied with the needs of others is simply confused about who needs whom.

162

The Dutiful Parent

Undeniably, the human infant would perish without care, but it does not follow that the relationship between parent and child is founded on a sense of obligation. As discussed in the last chapter, parents have their own reasons for wanting to care for their children, ranging from a desire to re-create and relive their own childhood to the healthier desire to see what manner of parents they can be. Why then speak of obligation to children? If people want to do something in any event, it is clearly gratuitous to insist that they feel obligated to do it.

It may be argued that the parent who for some reason lacks a desire to care for his child must be made to feel obligated to do so. But this is to overlook the fact that a person may or may not choose to fulfill an obligation. Unless he wants to do so, he will not act —barring coercion. And if coercion must be applied, the feeling of obligation is patently an ineffective motive.

Our concern here, however, is not with the rare parent who abandons his child, but rather with the typical American parent who feels obligated to do things for his children and thereby prevented from doing things for himself. For example, there is the father who feels obligated to take his children to the park, and has a sense of giving up things he would rather be doing. He may grumble, or he may go with a sense of self-sacrifice and a determined smile. But if he really did not want to take the children to the park he would find reason enough not to go. The simple fact is that, while he is ambivalent about it, his desire to go is stronger than his desire not to go, or he would not be there pushing the swing. But he has alienated his desire to take his children to the park and experiences it only as an obligation. *Duty or obligation is alienated desire. It is "I want to" rationalized as "I should."*

Turning desire into duty has some unfortunate consequences for the relationship between parent and child. The parent who feels obligated almost inevitably feels resentful about the trip to the park, the cost of the bicycle, or whatever the demand on his time and purse may be. Having lost sight of his desire to do or to give, he demands that the child appreciate the sacrifice he has made. Since the "sacrifice" was something the parent wanted to do, it is not at all clear why he merits gratitude, and it is certain that much of the time he will not receive it.

Moreover, the parent who transforms his desire to do something for his child into an obligation thereby precludes any evaluation of this desire. It becomes something he ought to do, and that the child ought to appreciate. The father who organizes a baseball team for a son with little interest in baseball is likely to proclaim in a martyred tone that his son does not appreciate the time and effort expended. Were he to recognize his own desire, he could evaluate it. He might then debate whether or not it was a good idea to act on his urge to organize a baseball team for his own son, but he is unlikely to ponder the wisdom of the move once he regards it as an obligation.

A sense of duty does not lead a parent to help his child in ways that he would not otherwise choose; rather, it leads him to enjoy less the things he wants to do with his child, and to be less sensible in his evaluation of these things.

The Dutiful Daughter

Typically, Americans regard their aged relatives with less veneration than most other peoples do. Still, the belief that parents of advanced years are the responsibility of their children has not disappeared from American culture; social security and pensions do not replace the emotional bond between parent and child, and Americans commonly feel that they "ought" to see more of their parents than they do. *But the statement "Mother needs me" is more accurately read backward.*

In its extreme form, this misunderstood motive characterizes the person who never marries at all, but devotes his life to his parents. In every town there is at least one, like the woman who had hoped to become a concert pianist but gave up her dream of studying in Europe to care for her ailing mother. For years she made a modest living giving piano lessons and playing for weddings and funerals. After her mother died, it seemed too late for the daughter to launch a career, but not too late for the trip to Europe, and her small inheritance and savings justified a summer tour. Friends assured her that after a life of self-sacrifice she owed herself the trip. But, before her plans became more than an inspection of travel brochures, she discovered a semi-invalid aunt who needed her. For some years now, she has been caring for her aunt and giving piano lessons.

This woman sacrificed herself not to duty, but to fear. Bluntly stated, she was afraid to leave her mother. Her self-doubts were so overwhelming that she was unwilling to venture beyond the shelter of her mother's home, or to assume responsibility for her own actions. The few decisions that she made were tentative arrangements, pending the invariable "talk with Mother."

It would have been difficult for her to accept the fact that she wanted to stay forever a child in her mother's home. But by alienating and projecting this desire onto her mother she could interpret it as her mother's need. Thus her desire became duty. Although her mother was by no means bedridden, "failing health" was a sufficient peg on which to hang the rationalization.

The concert career that might have been, acquired increasing promise in retrospect. Her acquaintances (mostly friends of her mother) lamented that her talent had to be sacrificed, and asked her to play for their daughters' weddings. Without putting her ability to the tests she feared, she could pretend that she had turned aside from a promising career to undertake the humble tasks of duty. In the small world bordering her mother's home, there was no one to challenge her rationalization. (This woman's counterpart is the dutiful mother who has similarly "sacrificed" a career to devote her life to her children.)

Self-doubts are not diminished by rationalization. When her mother died, this dedicated daughter felt lost. She enjoyed having friends say that she had earned a vacation, but she was terrified at the prospect of venturing into a strange city, and a foreign one at that. With unaccustomed initiative, she sought a new duty.

Obligation may thus mask a flight from life. More typically, the adjusted American assumes that because he is an adult he no longer needs his parents. But the parent remains an emotionally significant other for his child, regardless of age. When the adult experiences a desire to be with his parents, he typically reverses its direction and feels that his parents need him. Yet *dutifully* going to see them inhibits the warm interaction they all need.

The Dutiful Spouse

The sense of duty to one's spouse involves the same pattern of alienation as the sense of duty to parents and children. Perhaps the most common example is the wife who projects her sexual interests onto her husband and then dutifully submits to his desire. If he seeks a more enthusiastic bedmate, she is likely to say in bewilderment, "But I never refused him!"

The American husband typically feels a sense of obligation to provide for his wife, and at times the obligation can seem quite a burden. There is, for example, the husband who tries to be a good provider but feels that his wife is never satisfied. She needles him about the inadequacy of his income and insists on indulging expensive tastes. He sees his debts mount until he is convinced that if he lost a month's income he would be wiped out financially.

Being a good provider is typically a major element in the self-image of an American male, and it is an unusually strong part of this man's self-image. He wants to be the kind of man who can afford to give his family the best (the shade of Veblen would mutter something about "vicarious consumption by dependents" with "resulting increment of good repute to their master or patron"). Moreover, because this man loves his wife and children, he wants to take good care of the alienated facets of himself that he has hung on them to love. And in the home where he grew up, taking care of a family was understood in a material sense.

Thus he has a strong desire to provide expensive clothes, a suburban estate, vacations at exclusive resorts, and anything else that money can buy. But at the same time he is aware of his financial limitations. Because his own inclination to spend lavishly seems threatening to him, he projects it onto his wife. The projection fits, largely because he chose to marry a girl who expected the things he wanted to provide.

This man believes he is caught between his sense

of obligation and his resentment of his wife's demands. But he is actually caught between his desire to provide lavishly for his spouse (an expression of his neurotic quest for indirect self-acceptance) and his fear of bankruptcy (which to him symbolizes total inadequacy). If he ceased projecting his desire to indulge his wife, he could view her demands objectively, fulfilling them when possible and refusing them when they were unreasonable. His emotional turmoil reflects the internal nature of his conflict. So long as he feels torn between obligation and resentment, he *will* be trapped, for he cannot weigh and choose between his ambivalent desires when one side is alienated and regarded as a duty.

Sometimes a sense of duty masks a desire to keep the spouse helpless and dependent. Such motives are frequently encountered in the man who projects a desire to be dependent onto his wife. But it also occurs among women. A young woman married "for better, for worse" with full knowledge that she was marrying an alcoholic. Her family opposed the marriage, friends tried to dissuade her, but to no avail. She understood the problems and prognosis of alcoholism, she was aware that her husband would go on periodic binges, would have difficulty holding a job, would require at least occasional institutionalization, but she was adamant: "He needs me and I love him." And she married him, proclaiming that her husband was a man of rare ability who needed someone to have faith in him, to help reclaim his life. True to her culture, she believed that love could conquer any obstacle, alcoholism included.

What this woman loved in her husband was her own dependent, irresponsible, and self-destructive desires, which she had projected onto him. Moreover, she needed faith in herself and wanted someone to bring out the best in her. These needs, too, she projected onto her alcoholic husband, where she ministered to them tenderly.

Moreover, if he had not so obviously needed someone to take care of him, she would have feared that he might lose interest in her. Although a woman of potential charm, her self-image was unrealistically negative. Uncertain of her ability to hold a husband, she married a man who would be tied to her by his needs. Had his prognosis been more favorable, she would have felt less secure. What neither the woman nor her family recognized was that she loved her husband because he was an alcoholic, not in spite of the fact. But she was unwilling to acknowledge her desire to have her husband dependent on her, and turned it into a loving duty.

The Minor Duties

A desire to do something is very likely to be interpreted as an obligation if the individual can see no reason why he would *want* to do it. This is particularly likely to be the case when the desire springs from the need to validate the self-image, rather than from some intrinsic reward in the action.

Suppose a man makes it a custom to take his aging aunt (a prepossessing dowager) for a Sunday afternoon drive. This consumes most of the afternoon, as staying for tea is part of the weekly ritual. There are usually any number of things he would rather do on Sunday afternoon, but he is certain that the drive means a lot to her and so he goes to discharge his duty.

It is difficult for him to see any reason why he would want to keep his Sunday date with his aunt, but he has at least two motives. First, his self-image includes being the sort of fellow who is kind to elderly relatives. But not thinking of the contribution it makes to his good opinion of himself, he assumes that he is kind to her out of a sense of obligation.

The second motive is the hope that he will be fondly remembered in her will. This is a desire he could find plausible enough if he were not ashamed to admit it, but he projects it onto his grasping cousin. By assuming that he sees his aunt out of duty, he avoids recognition of this motive.

But having alienated his desire to visit his aunt, he is conscious only of the side of his ambivalence that would rather do something else. If he could recognize that he does have reasons of his own for wanting to see her, he would be able to find more enjoyment in his visits. Moreover, he could feel free to cancel the drive on occasion. Finally, the will would not seem such an ignoble interest if he recognized that he had another motive for seeing his aunt.

But, lacking insight, this man is not likely to inquire into his motives—or into the possibility that his aunt may find the dutiful visits of a bored nephew rather tiresome.

Beyond Obligation

Duty is but the mirror image of desire. It is a neurotic rationalization of the individual's own wishes. But, judging others by his own confusion, the adjusted American is likely to argue that if everyone perceived that duty is a myth, society would collapse. Yet people are hardly less likely to assume responsibilities if they recognize their desire to do so. Quite the contrary, it is the desire which alienation transforms into obligation that men perform perfunctorily, or evade altogether.

In American culture, something done for others is regarded as more worthy than something done for oneself. Doing only what one wants to do is considered selfish. Yet people do what they most want to do, often justifying it by calling it their duty. People are motivated by their own needs. As each man seeks to find himself acceptable and to exercise his capacity for warm, intimate association, he is likely to engage in acts of kindness, generosity, and the like. But his motive is his own need; *he does not do things for others—rather, others are the recipients of actions he engages in for himself.*

Even in moralistic categories, it may be most selfish to expect gratitude from someone else for acting on one's own desire—even when the other person happens to benefit from the action. It is rather like expecting gratitude from the poor for attending a charity ball.

13
UNDER PRESSURE

Now here [said the Red Queen] it takes all the running you can do to keep in the same place. If you want to get somewhere else, you must run at least twice as fast as that! LEWIS CARROLL

The sense of pressure in American life is often remarked by foreign visitors, who feel, like Alice, that it is a queer country where the inhabitants run as hard as they can in order to hold their own. It seems particularly queer in a country where the standard of living is so bounteous and the apparatus for leisure activity so highly elaborated. Yet growing affluence and increasing opportunities for leisure have done little to diminish the American's feeling of being under pressure; being an official in a sailing club or chairman of the community chest drive seldom seems to reduce the individual's level of tension. Especially to Americans in the upper-middle classes, it often seems that among job, family, and community activities, at least thirty hours a day are firmly committed.

The urban (and suburban) American tends to assume that the pressures he feels are an inevitable by-product of modern urban life and that the only escape would lie in a retreat to a rural existence. Implicit in this view is the notion that the economic necessities of rural life do not entail the kinds of pressure which trouble the urbanite. Hard work in a country setting is supposed to bring a unique sense of fulfillment.

Obviously, this idyllic view of rural life has not resulted in a mass migration back to the farm. However, a rapidly growing number of urban Americans do retreat to a weekend cottage in the mountains or a summer place along some rocky coast. Most of these people claim to be seeking escape from pressure, yet apparently they are not dismayed by an endless number of things to be done to maintain their property and themselves. Their behavior is not inconsistent, it is instructive. The man painting his cottage or calking his boat has escaped the sense of continuous pressure from other people. Apparently the irritant is the feeling of being under pressure from others, not the amount to be done.

In large measure, the sense of being under pressure is a result of the quest for indirect self-acceptance. As the adjusted American is caught up in this misdirected pursuit, most of what he does is undertaken for the effect it will have on other people. Thus he imposes on himself a constant concern with what he thinks other people think he should be doing, or how other people evaluate what he has done. Such misplaced concern underlies his sense of an endless striving leading nowhere—which is approximately where his efforts do lead. No matter how hard he works at it, he will never arrive at *self*-acceptance by doing things to impress other people.

Moreover, so long as he expends his energy in this fruitless quest, he will remain unsatisfied and tense. The American is prone to misinterpret this tension—which arises from his unfilled needs—and to regard it as anger, anxiety, and pressure. Believing that what he wants is success, high status, popularity, or prestige, he pursues these things, but the pressure never eases.

As Fromm has observed, "It is in the very nature of irrational desires that they cannot be 'satisfied.' They spring from a dissatisfaction within oneself." [1] This neurotic pattern has been discussed at length in chapter 6. We bring it up again at this point because a major component of what the American regards as pressure is actually a by-product of the neurotic quest for indirect self-acceptance.

Another major factor contributing to the sense of pressure from others is the tendency for the individual to lose sight of his own drive. Projecting his drive onto someone else, he believes that what he feels is pressure emanating from that person. If he acts on his projected drive it seems to him that he is knuckling under to pressure, yet if he refuses to act on it he is left with a disquieting anxiety. Having made the projection he cannot make a valid assessment of his ambivalent desires. This neurotic pattern is normal among Americans, and the following examples illustrate some of the many forms it can take.

Paved with Good Intentions

In a house down the street there is a man and a garage. It is Saturday morning, and the man feels that he should straighten the garage. The thought has been in his mind for some weeks, and he has taken to closing the garage door quickly. By now the task has assumed Herculean proportions and seems akin to cleaning the Augean stables. He sits in his chair, glances over the morning paper for the second time, and worries about the garage.

It would never occur to some men to straighten a garage, far less to worry about it. Neatness is not a significant part of every man's self-image. This particular man, however, is appalled by the mess. Yet, shifting in his chair, he begins to read the paper for the third time.

Refusing to act on his alienated drive is an exhausting process. His unacknowledged desire to get the job done is strong enough that he cannot simply drop it and do something else, so he sits and struggles with it. Feeling at once tense and enervated, he tries to get comfortable and to distract himself with the well-thumbed financial page.

Enter his wife, with the suggestion that since he apparently has nothing else to do this morning he might clean the garage. Now a man innocent of any urge to do so might either ignore or view with amazement such a suggestion from wife. But this man leaps at her remark with something akin to relief—*she* wants him to clean the garage! He declares heatedly that he has worked hard all week, that it is unreasonable to expect him to clean the garage today, and that if he is not allowed peace at home he will spend his Saturday's elsewhere.

But finally, though still muttering about a man's right to relax, he attacks the garage. To his surprise, he feels exhilarated as he digs out the first layer. He has to admit that it was harder to worry about the garage than to clean it; that is to say, *it took more energy to fight his alienated drive than to act on it.* As a kind of bonus, he finds an old jacket he had thought lost. Feeling immensely pleased with himself, he makes great resolves for future order. But the odds are that he will go through the same struggle again toward the end of the year.

Like this man, most Americans project many of their own drives simply because they cannot imagine having them. Every person requires diverse physical and mental activity in order to experience his many capacities, and thus potentially can find almost any activity rewarding. Yet every person acquires ambivalent attitudes toward most actions. Not having learned to expect ambivalence, he is likely to alienate his interest in doing many things. He is most likely to alienate his interest in doing the things he labels "work," which unfortunately includes most of his activities. (Significant exceptions are found among individuals who are financially able to live without "working," and are often quite conscious of their need for purposeful activity.)

The more routine the activity, the more likely it is to be considered an unwanted task. Thus most housewives are annoyed or amused (depending on their temperament) when the pitchman suggests that his non-soap will make dishwashing *almost* fun. But to ask the seemingly foolish question, why is dishwashing *not* fun? There is nothing intrinsically unpleasant about the task, as every little girl who has washed her doll's dishes in the bathtub knows. If her family is typical, however, the little girl's mother regards dishwashing as a chore and as soon as the child is old enough to be useful is likely to say, "The least you can do is help wash the dishes." Daughter gets the point. She learns to enjoy the tea party, but to alienate her interest in washing the dishes.

The person who grumbles most about a particular chore usually spends more time at it than other people do. He obviously does not want to be the sort of person who neglects the job, for if it did not matter to his self-image he could simply walk off and leave it undone. Yet, failing to perceive his reason for wanting to undertake the task, he does not let himself enjoy it. The ensuing struggle to get the job done in spite of himself is time-consuming and unrewarding.

A routine activity is almost by definition one which the individual spends a good deal of his life doing.

He thus has a considerable interest in getting as much pleasure from it as he can. That most activities can be enjoyed is evident from the fact that one man's work is another man's recreation: gardening, carpentry, overhauling an old automobile, breeding cattle, deep-sea fishing. Whether an activity is work or play depends on the point of view. The importance of perspective is unforgettably illustrated by the whitewashing of Tom Sawyer's fence.

The Path to Promotion

Sometimes it is not so much that a person fails to enjoy the things he does as that he thinks he has an impossible amount to do. Picture a professor returned home from an evening seminar, settled into his favorite chair, and thinking about a research report he feels he should be writing. He has had a long day, in which two undergraduate classes were a prelude to preparing a lecture, lab work, a frustrating committee meeting, a student with thesis problems, and (after a hurried dinner) a three-hour graduate seminar. It seems to him that he has done a day's work by any reasonable standard and that the research report could wait until tomorrow.

Tomorrow will bring its own problems, however, and his university is one of those referred to by faculty as a "pressure cooker," where publish or perish is the rule. He has to maintain a steady output of published research if he wants to be promoted. But when he thinks wistfully of his neighbors watching television and wonders how it would feel to be out from under pressure, he tends to forget that he knew what he was getting into when he was in graduate school. Moreover, he could have taken a job in industry and worked only a forty-hour week at a higher salary. He could still do so. But, although he likes to mull on this possibility when feeling imposed on by the university administration, the truth is that he chose his profession and likes it well enough to stay with it.

The pressure that lies most heavily upon him is his own drive. He is ambitious. His self-image involves achieving national standing in his field and, moreover, he enjoys research (a fact he *sometimes* recognizes). In addition he really likes to teach; he finds his students rewarding, he does far more counseling than his job requires, and spends more time preparing lectures than do most of his colleagues. Being the kind of teacher he wants to be is a full-time job and, when the research he wants to do is added, his combined objectives *are* demanding.

Inevitably he is ambivalent about the pace he has set. He makes excessive demands on himself and at the same time thinks longingly of leisure. Aware that the demands on his time are unreasonable, he finds it implausible that he would inflict them on himself and tends to think of them as emanating from the university administration. The administration invites the projection, for it does give raises and promotions most readily to those who publish frequently (or are able to secure lucrative foundation grants).

But in his grumbling about the administration this professor overlooks the possibility of taking a job at one of the many schools that do not make publication the basis for promotion. This is a deliberate oversight; although he may prefer to ignore the fact, he chooses to teach at a university that *will* put pressure on him. He is competent, but knows that many of his colleagues are equally competent, and he feels that he can get ahead only as a result of drive and application. He fears that without external pressure he would slow down into mediocrity. This fear has led him to seek out the very pressure he resents.

Having projected most of his own drive, he is disproportionately aware of his desire to slow down. This desire then becomes a problem to him. It can seem to be a debilitating lethargy, a dead weight that he must drag along. Yet at the same time he tends to see this desire to slow down as what he really wants to do, rather than as the counterpoise to his drive. The projection of his drive interferes with both his work and his leisure, for he spends more time than he realizes in the unproductive and unenjoyable state of doing nothing because he can neither make himself work nor let himself play.

Do It for Mother

Experiencing one's own drive as if it were unwelcome external pressure is a prevalent pattern among Americans. In large measure this is a result of the insistent way in which many American mothers usurp their children's needs and turn them into parental dictates. The tiny child is wheedled or commanded to take a bite for mother or to drink his milk for father. He soon acquires the notion that these are things he does for other people, rather than for himself. The result is a child who picks over his food at meals, feeling not hungry but pressured. He remains capable of recognizing his hunger well enough between meals, however, and as soon as he is old enough to clutch a dime and run he will be pursuing the ice cream truck down the street.

The same pattern of interaction leads the child to alienate his desire to curl up and sleep when he is tired. Going to sleep becomes something he does to please his mother. If he is in no mood to please his mother, naptime and bedtime become a contest of wills. Similarly, when and where he relieves himself are matters subject to parental pressure long before he is able to talk. Indeed, most of the American child's basic physiological needs—eating, sleeping, defecating, urinating—are likely to become things which his parents insist that he do.

Thus the child it taught to alienate his needs and to experience them as external pressures, emanating from his parents. Hunger, thirst, fatigue, and other inner drives are supplemented—and at the conscious level often supplanted—by a desire to win praise or to avoid punishment. The threat that most frequently hangs over the child is the withdrawal of parental love. The child may eat, not because he feels hungry but because he is afraid his mother may not love him if he refuses his food. Once the child has been made emotionally dependent on the love of his parents (as discussed in chapter 11), this dependence becomes a point of leverage from which the child can be manipulated.

Sooner or later the child is likely to rebel against parental imperatives and to be caught up in a battle for control. Suppose a small girl refuses her carrots at one meal only to find nothing but warmed-over carrots served to her at the next. She is faced with a dilemma. She can submit to parental pressure at once, or she can go on a hunger strike. If she gives in at once and the pattern is repeated, the result is a "good" child who will submit readily to pressures applied by Authority, a child who will become an equally submissive adult.

On the other hand, if the little girl goes on a hunger strike she is openly challenging Authority. Her mother may not only keep on reheating the carrots, she will also be very likely to let her daughter know that no one loves a child who refuses to eat her nice carrots. If the girl gives in and ingests the despised vegetable, she will have eaten a good deal of humble pie besides. Again, she will have made a large step toward becoming a submissive conformist who does distasteful things because people insist that she must, and will not like her if she refuses.

If the mother gives in first, she will be likely to feel that she has done much more than dump a plate of warmed-over carrots down the garbage disposer. She will feel that her very authority over the child has been weakened. Her self-image as a parent will be threatened. At the next opportunity she will try to reassert her authority, and a return battle of wills will be waged. If the child had been left to satisfy her hunger or allowed the simple dignity of refusing something that she did not at that moment want, there would never have been an issue. But because the mother preempted the child's needs, such a simple thing as food has become a point of friction between parent and child.

The next stage is likely to be a running battle over such things as piano lessons. Here is the little girl who is deaf to parental prophecies that someday she will regret her refusal to practice. She can be made to sit on the piano bench but not to learn. The piano lessons were initiated because she liked to pick out tunes, and at first she was thrilled with learning. But the other side of her ambivalence soon emerged as her aspirations outran her ability. Nevertheless, she has a lingering desire to play the piano and if left alone would practice more often than not.

But she is not left alone. Her mother sees practice as a means to the distant goal of playing well, and the idea that practice itself could be rewarding has never occurred to her. She communicates this feeling to the child at the same time that she pressures her daughter to practice. The girl is thus encouraged to take a negative view of the learning process and to project her interest in music onto her mother. Having alienated her desire to play the piano, she is conscious only of her distaste for finger exercises.

Some children who have hung similar projections on their parents comply with the pressure. This little girl is stubborn. She has a pervasive sense of parental pressure to do things (having projected most of her desires and drives onto her mother) and wants to prove that she is not completely cowed. Inevitably she submits sooner or later to her mother's insistence in such matters as eating, sleeping, and defecating, but she can flatly refuse to play the piano. Taking a stand on the issue becomes a symbolic mutiny. Eventually her mother's reiterated comments on the child's stubborn streak enter her self-image as something in which she takes a defiant pride.

Moreover, her refusal to practice may be a means of testing her mother's affection. Without really formulating the thought, she may wonder if her mother would still like her if she refused to practice at all (unlike some of the "good" girls to whom her mother compares her, she apparently feels secure enough in her mother's affection to make the test).

The pressure which the mother applies is motivated in large measure by her own desire to play the piano. She feels she is giving her child an opportunity which she herself was denied; in reality she is trying to live vicariously through her child. She scoffs when an insightful friend suggests that perhaps she might enroll with the piano teacher herself, but suppose that after a stormy session with her daughter she acted on the suggestion. Given the mother's level of motivation (and an added fillip of spite) she would probably progress rapidly.

Daughter would then be left with her projections dangling. She would feel *someone* wanting her to play the piano, but her mother would be increasingly indifferent to whether the girl practiced or not. After a period of experimenting with the idea that perhaps her father wanted her to take piano lessons, the child would begin to recognize her own interest. For some time, the slightest pressure from either parent would invite her to project and rebel again, but in the end mother and daughter could act independently on their respective desires to play.

Black Sheep

The person who is hanging between two courses of action may not be at all sure which he wants to take until someone brings pressure to bear in favor of one or against the other. With this invitation to project one side of his ambivalence, the individual quickly loses sight of his own desire and experiences it as external pressure. The other course of action is suddenly the only one he is aware of wanting to take. What was a choice between alternative actions thus becomes an apparent choice between defiance or submission.

This pattern is particularly common between an adolescent and his parents. Suppose that a high school girl becomes interested in a boy who is decidedly not the type of young man her family has in mind for her. Her parents cannot understand what she sees in him. Quite simply, what she sees is alienated sides of herself. Suppose the boy is rough, slovenly, insolent, and reckless—he will be an excellent target for the alienated potential which her antiseptically middle-class background has made both frightening and fascinating. Suppose, moreover, that he treats her as a sexually attractive woman and thus offers her an image of herself which she covets—and fears. When she met him she was torn between attraction and revulsion. But her father formed an instant dislike for the boy (making about the same projections on him that his daughter does, he responds with indignation). The father forbids his daughter to see the boy again. Predictably, she falls in love. With some variations, this is the theme of numerous movies (perhaps most memorably *The Wild One*).

Such a girl is attracted to alienated sides of herself which she experiences only with her boy friend, and which are the more exciting because they are forbidden. Her own desire to break off the relationship is projected and experienced as if it were parental pressure to do so. Added to the pressure which *is* emanating from that quarter, it seems intolerable coercion. She balks, then rebels. Once it becomes evident that she intends to defy her parents, they could dissolve the romance sooner by ignoring it than by forbidding it. But this is a little late to alter a pattern of pressure and defiance that probably goes back to eating her vegetables and taking her nap.

Some people chronically project their desire to take one course of action rather than another, and become preoccupied with defying attitudes that are in reality their own. They may even build their lives around such defiance. For example, a rigidly puritanical family is likely to have a Drinking Uncle who drinks not so much for pleasure as for principle. He resists all of the pressures his relatives exert to help him abandon his vice, even weathering the expensive cure that his family once imposed on him. Repeated family councils have only reaffirmed everyone's disapproval. Uncle keeps on coming to family gatherings with whiskey on his breath.

Like the other members of his family, the Drinking Uncle was raised to regard alcohol as an instrument of the Devil. Like the others, he is ambivalent. He differs from the rest in that he has alienated his desire to live a life of abstinence, and regards it as pressure from his relatives to do so. (He is encouraged in the projection by the pressures they do try to apply.) Most other members of the clan have in turn alienated their desire to sample the demon rum and have projected it onto Uncle (who in turn invites this projection).

What Uncle does (and thus what he has become in the course of time) is determined largely by defiance of pressure. Yet he could view the attitudes of his relatives with detachment. When he shocks his family he is actually striking at the alienated teetotaler in himself.

Defiance of pressure is a pattern of behavior he learned at his mother's knee. When he was a small boy, his mother would call him aside and lecture him about being polite when Auntie Dear arrived. Projecting her own desire to greet that prim soul with a loud raspberry, she was quite explicit about what the little boy was not to do. With the idea of being rude—and specific suggestions about how to be rude—planted in his mind, he at once perceived the situation as a challenge. Was he or was he not going to be intimidated by his mother and kissed by his aunt? With a a sense of asserting his budding manhood, he was horrid.

Over the years, shocking his relatives has become a matter of principle, and defying the pressures he believes they exert has become an end in itself. As an adult he finds that being horrid means listing slightly as he enters the room and giving elderly Auntie Dear a bleary-eyed wink.

Beyond Pressure

The adjusted American has learned to interpret most of his own drive as if it were external pressure, and the result is that he feels under pressure most of the time. He may defy what he believes to be pressure from others. But even if he complies with it he is likely to put up a good deal of resistance, and his enjoyment and efficiency both ebb. The things he believes are expected of him seem to stretch endlessly before him, and he may become so dispirited as to believe that he requires external pressure in order to accomplish anything at all—here is the final turn of the screw.

With much of his energy diverted to a struggle against his own drive, he has a sense of running as hard as he can but with little progress to show for his effort. Considering the amount of internal resistance he has to overcome before he moves, perhaps it is remarkable that there is any progress at all.

The autonomous alternative is to move beyond pressure by recognizing that any sense of insistent pressure is one's own projected drive. The man who recognizes that what he feels is his own drive will neither resent nor resist the pressure; he will act.

It is sometimes difficult for the individual to credit the intensity of his own drive. Yet the intensity should not be surprising, for the source of man's drive to action lies in basic human needs. In order to be acceptable in his own eyes, a man must act as he believes an acceptable person would act. He must use all of the many capacities he values in himself, for disuse of any capacity, like disuse of a muscle, leads to atrophy. And he has a continuing need to discover and experience what he is through what he does. Thus, in the final analysis, the only escape from pressure lies in affirming the drive to action.

14

BARRIERS
AND RESTRAINTS

What is an obstacle for me may not be so for another. There is no obstacle in an absolute sense. . . . Human-reality everywhere encounters resistance and obstacles which it has not created, but these resistances and obstacles have meaning only in and through the free choice which human-reality is. JEAN-PAUL SARTRE

There is a story about a drunk who left his favorite bar, pulled his eyes into focus, and charted his homeward course. At the corner he collided with a lamppost. Staggering back a few steps, he took his bearings and then advanced on the same collision course. Inevitably he struck and this time he fell. But he gathered himself up with patient resolution and retraced his steps once more. Colliding with the lamppost again, he clung to it and sobbed in defeat, "It's no use, I'm fenced in."

The feeling of being surrounded by obstacles is familiar to the adjusted American. Yet, like the drunk, he is fenced in primarily by his own confusion. This is not to say that obstacles exist solely in the mind—many of them are real enough, but then the lamppost was no illusion either. It is not that people hallucinate obstacles but rather that they fail to veer around them.

Those who argue that obstacles are often insurmountable are fond of citing extreme cases—double amputees or prisoners in solitary confinement—but the fact remains that in normal life there are few obstacles which are in themselves capable of blocking fulfillment of the individual. His cooperation, witting or unwitting, is required.

Particularization

The adjusted American often allows obstacles to thwart him because he has only a particularized understanding of his needs. Human needs are broad and can be satisfied in a variety of ways. But the person who is blinded by habit and by the conventional assumptions of this culture perceives not his need but only his customary and highly particular means of satisfying it. If he encounters an obstacle to this particular avenue of satisfaction, he feels trapped. Because his perception is limited to one single approach, he can only collide with the obstacle, retrace his steps, and collide again. In the end he may admit defeat, or he may assert hopefully that a bloody head is a sign of progress.

This mechanism is often involved in the major crises of life, as when a man feels that the loss of a loved one has robbed him of all meaningful association, that retirement is an insurmountable barrier to purposeful activity, or that a crushing defeat has forever shattered his self-acceptance. Folk wisdom asserts that time will heal such wounds—which is another way of saying that after the initial period of stunned deprivation most people are able to find alternative means of satisfying these basic needs.

Although most people are able to weather a major crisis, few deal effectively with the trivial frustrations of daily life. The latter are taken for granted as inevitable irritants, more stumbling blocks than barriers. Yet, taken in the aggregate, the daily collisions with minor obstacles may bruise a man's spirit and abrade his enjoyment of life more than the occasional crisis. And quite unnecessarily so, in view of the relative ease with which he could step around or leap over such stumbling blocks.

The person caught up in particularization may be deprived simply for want of the capacity to perceive —or to accept—alternatives. He may be aware that other people find other ways to satisfy their needs, yet feel that only the familiar ones will satisfy *him*. As long as his habitual patterns of life are even marginally feasible, he will stay doggedly in his particular rut. Consequently, he stays lined up with the obstacles in his old rut, when he could be exploring new approaches.

The sullen inaction called boredom is an example of this pattern. Imagine a bored adolescent vacationing with his parents, away from his usual companions, haunts, and activities. To an objective observer, the resort town offers endless possibilities for rewarding activity: hills to be climbed, water sports, tennis courts, even drive-in movies and other adolescents. But to this boy the friends and familiar pastimes at home seem the only interesting ones. He mopes around the hotel reading well-thumbed science fiction, and flares into open anger at the slightest pretext. The usual path to satisfaction is blocked, and he refuses to consider any other.

Particularization is not the only reason he fails to seek new avenues of satisfaction; he does nothing interesting because he chooses to be miserable in order to punish his parents for making him miserable. By not having a good time, he seeks to prove that he was right when he predicted that the vacation would be a "drag." He refuses to try water skiing, partly because he suspects that he might have fun. He believes that enjoying himself would be tantamount to admitting that his parents were right, and he prefers to sit and glower. The complaint that, "There is nothing to do" translates freely, "Damned if I'll do anything."

The Inhibited Life   *impecunious – habitually poor*

Some people find obstacles insurmountable largely because they are confused about where they want to go. They may lament their inability to attain some bogus satisfaction, which would not fulfil them if they achieved it, while ignoring the many approaches to fulfillment that are open to them. Thus the adjusted American sharply limits himself as he pursues indirect self-acceptance. Focused on this bogus satisfaction, he is concerned not with doing, but with impressing. When he laments that he cannot do something, what he usually means is that he cannot do it grandly.

This point is nowhere more clearly exemplified than in the obstacle bemoaned by Americans of every income level—lack of money. There is no denying the utility of money, but it is less omnipotent and less necessary than most Americans assume. The impecunious find specific avenues blocked, but the more ingenious among them find other means to their ends.

To take one example, people with limited means and a desire to travel have hitchiked, built sailboats in the back yard, and at least one couple we know of worked their way around the world as a short-order cook and waitress. The person who says that he longs to travel but is financially unable to do so usually has in mind first-class travel by jet, and is less interested in the trip than in the illustrated lecture he could give to his service club after he returned.

Lack of funds may be an inconvenience, but hardly an insurmountable barrier for most Americans. What seems to be a money problem is usually a disguised problem of self-acceptance. Except for the truly impoverished minority, the people who claim that lack of funds prevents them from doing something are focused on the prestige value of having the money (or credit) to do it, and not on the activity at all. What they seek is a way to indirect self-acceptance— in this instance, the glitter of money to enhance an otherwise unimposing self-image. In a culture where price has long been considered the most reliable index of quality, it is not surprising that people try to inflate their financial worth when seeking indirect self-acceptance. Having the conviction that money is the solution to all problems, the American cannot quite get it through his head that money cannot buy self-esteem.

In a similar vein, lack of talent seldom presents a real barrier to activity. Some people who are quite patently tone-deaf nonetheless find a great deal of satisfaction in singing, making up in verve what they lick in pitch. The person who demurs, pleading lack of ability, is focused on the judgment others may pass on his efforts, not on his own potential enjoyment. He is envious of the praise that the accomplished artist receives, and terrified that he would be a laughingstock if he ventured to try. His perception of his capacities is distorted by his quest for indirect self-acceptance. He is inhibited by fear of failure, not by a total lack of capacity. It is not that he cannot, but rather that he cannot excel.

Thus there is a woman who envies the ability of

her neighbor, a commercial artist. The artist uses her children and their friends as models, and the woman often follows her little girl to her neighbor's studio. This woman is fascinated by seeing a drawing take form under her neighbor's skillful fingers. The children who watch usually want to draw, too, and the artist provides them with paper and colored chalk. The childish sketches often have one eye higher than the other and arms that seem to be in splints, but they have charm, and the children execute them with pleasure. The woman finds herself watching the children with interest too, yet, when offered paper and chalk, she turns them down with an embarrassed laugh and an emphatic, "I can't draw!"

What she means, of course, is that she cannot draw as well as the trained artist, and is afraid of making a fool of herself if she tried. The children have no such fears; they enjoy watching but they enjoy drawing more, and they make no invidious comparisons with the professional.

A child wants to try everything, enjoys himself in the process, and likes the finished product because he made it. But if he embarks on the quest for indirect self-acceptance (as the adjusted American child soon does), he begins to do things for the impression he can make on others ("showing off" is the colloquial phrase) and gradually loses the direct pleasure of the activity. By the time he is an adult, he has learned to hang back in areas where he lacks natural gifts or previous training.

His desire to try something turns to envy of those who can do it superbly. Along with millions of his fellows, he becomes only an admiring spectator. But there is a pleasure in doing, in developing and exercising self-potential, that no amount of vicarious participation can simulate. Moreover, the person who has learned the rudiments of an art (or a sport) finds the artistry of a master more exciting, for he understands and appreciates the difficulty of technique, the nuance of expression. In contrast, the person who has never been more than a passive spectator is not even capable of being a responsive audience for the artist. He can grasp only the most superficial and obvious elements of a performance which is totally outside his own experience.

The Tar Baby

The Uncle Remus tale made it abundantly clear that the advisable way to deal with tar babies is to by-pass, or cautiously to remove them, not to assault them headlong. The point of the parable of the stag and the brambles in chapter 2 was essentially the same. But in the conflicts of life this point is easily forgotten. The person who encounters an obstacle can become so focused on removing it that destruction of the obstacle becomes an end in itself, rather than a means of reaching his original goal.

A not uncommon example is the junior executive whose immediate superior is incompetent and tyrannical. To the young man, it seems that advancement in his career and enjoyment of his work are impossible under such circumstances. He becomes preoccupied with the shortcomings of his boss. With his attention fixed on the obstacle, he develops what might be called mental tunnel vision, blocking perception of other routes to his goal and even of the goal itself. He does not seek to maximize the opportunities that (his superior notwithstanding) his job does offer, nor does he try to arrange a transfer to another branch of the company, nor look for another job. He does not even join in the quiet but persistent efforts of his colleagues to have the division manager replaced—he feels that his colleagues are not aggressive enough. Any one of these alternatives, or some combination of them, might have served his interests. But he chooses instead the one course of action least likely to accomplish his ends: a frontal assault on the "tar baby."

Hurling himself into office intrigue, he loses track of his desire to find satisfaction in his job; destruction of the immediate obstacle becomes an end in itself. It is probable that heads will ultimately roll, his among them. He may well find that he is dismissed as a troublemaker shortly before the manager is transferred—as a result of the quiet but persistent efforts of others.

The person engaged in such a self-defeating attack on an obstacle is blinded by a passion that he believes to be the fury of frustration. What he feels is in reality the mounting tension generated by unfilled needs but, interpreting his tension as anger at the people who seem to thwart him, he is led to assault the immediate obstacle.

Another person caught up in the same misunderstanding may regard his "anger" as dangerous or unreasonable, and instead of attacking the apparent obstacle may turn the "anger" back on himself. The resulting depression may well block any action at all. Instead of acting to meet his pressing need, he tries to dissipate his mounting tension. (At this point he may simply reach for the tranquilizers.)

Cherished Obstacles

There are some obstacles which people seek out and claim for their own. These are the external circumstances which they use to rationalize their self-doubts, and if such obstacles were suddenly to evaporate they would be panic-stricken. But if the obstacles are to serve the function for which they are valued, people must believe these barriers are not of their own choosing. To strengthen this illusion, they engage in a great deal of ritualistic griping about these cherished obstacles.

A typical example is the man who finds himself at middle age in a mediocre, blind-alley job and, suspecting that he has reached the pinnacle of his career, claims that the reason is his lack of a college education. Invariably, he can point to formidable external obstacles which kept him from college—the depression, the war, or early family responsibilities—ignoring the fact that similar obstacles have not deterred others. Over the years, such a man acquires an exaggerated image of the "college man," and, doubtful of his ability to measure up to this image, avoids every opportunity to take night classes or otherwise venture into the college classroom. He fears failure more than he wants an education.

Moreover, if he acquired an education he would have vitiated the principal rationalization with which he explains away his failures. When a coveted promotion goes to someone else, he consoles himself with the thought that the firm gives preference to college men, and tells himself that college men are not so deserving as a man who has had to struggle ahead without an education. By a reverse twist, his envy turns to suspicion. He is likely to be an outspoken anti-intellectual, and to overlook the fact that this is inconsistent with his reiterated complaint that he was denied a college education.

The obstacle to which an individual clings may be a set of circumstances, or it may be another person who appears to be blocking an action. Relying on the probability that some other person will exercise a restraining influence, people often find it exciting to pretend that they are seriously contemplating action which they would otherwise find frightening. Like a toy terrier straining his leash, a man may do a good deal of barking about things he would do if he were not held back. But the leash is actually a safety line.

There is, let us say, a man arranging his arguments on the 5:35. He has decided that tomorrow he will tell his boss what he thinks of him, what he thinks of company policy, and that he is resigning. He tells himself that he has taken all that his dignity permits, and although he knows his wife will protest, he has made up his mind. It should be noted that if he had serious intentions of making a scene at the office tomorrow he would be shivering with anxiety. He is not.

He is engaging in fantasy, yet it would cost him a good deal to admit the fact. He would like to be a lion, and he finds it easier to give credence to his leonine potential if he believes that it is firmly leashed by his wife's desire for security. (Besides, it is safer to roar at his wife than at his boss.) He is preparing to quash her objections—but in such a way that, without allowing himself to be aware of the process, he will suggest to her all of the arguments which she can use to restrain him.

This pattern is common among Americans, but perhaps least understood in the American adolescent. Many adolescents talk a wilder life than they have any inclination to live, secure in the knowledge that they can tug against (that is, cling to) parental restrictions. The anxious and troubled ones are the adolescents who have no clear lines drawn for them, who probe beyond the point where they are comfortable with themselves in an attempt to find what limits their parents may set if pressed hard enough.

Having no traditional pattern on which he can model himself, the American adolescent needs consistent parental expectations as a framework within which he can develop a conception of what he is and what he wants to be. If he encounters only erratic vacillation among indifference, indulgence, and indignation, he is forced to grope without direction toward a viable self-image. What appears to be a rebellion against his parents is often a search for reassuring restraint.

Projected Restraint

Many of the obstacles which the adjusted American encounters derive from the projection of his inner resistance to an undertaking. When he alienates his self-restraint, he becomes hyperconscious of the other side of his ambivalence. Having surrounded himself with projected self-restraint, he feels fenced in by prohibitions he attributes to others.

Here is the man who posts with morose conviction a wall placard that proclaims, "Everything I want to do is immoral, illegal, or fattening," then pencils in "or cancer inducing." At every turn his wife, his doctor, his minister, the police, and people in the broadening circle extending from "they" out to "society" seem joined in an effort to take the fun out of his life. Not that he sees it as a conspiracy directed against him; it is more that he feels he must stay within narrow limits designated by others. Someday, he promises himself, he will tell them all where to go and spend the rest of his life eating, smoking, wenching, and evading income tax.

He resents the limitations because he has lost sight of the fact that they are self-imposed. Having been told that he ought to refrain from certain activities, he has found it increasingly difficult to recognize that he wants to refrain. Yet he knows that there are people who break the law and find that crime pays well.

He knows people who patronize call girls and charge them to their expense accounts. Many of his acquaintances are chain smokers, apparently willing to take their chances on lung cancer, and few people he knows are as careful of calories and cholesterol as he is. Several of his friends have driven for years in a manner he contemplates with a mixture of envy and horror: one is dead and another out on bail, but the others remain unrepentent.

All of these people are subject to the same kind of external prohibitions that he is, and they are not deterred. He notes this fact, but with resentment and indignation rather than enlightenment. What he fails to perceive is that he is restrained by his own choice. In the long run, unpleasant consequences may follow from certain decisions, but at the moment of choice no external restraint short of iron manacles and a short chain can prevent him from doing largely as he pleases.

The idea that men are controlled by inner choice rather than by external coercion is threatening to some people. There are tormented souls who have magnified the side of their ambivalence which frightens them, and, having made it into a pseudo-monster, believe that they possess an urge to do evil that is too powerful to be checked by their will alone. The fact that it is their own counter-urge for restraint that has checked them all their lives is difficult for them to accept, for they have projected their inner restraint onto authority or Divinity. Until they recall their projections, they will be fearful that without external controls they would run amuck.

It is more common for people to fear the possible antisocial actions of others (that is, to project antisocial potential) and thus some will argue that so long as people think they are held back by external coercion they will behave as if they were. Why, then, disabuse them and run the risk of having them get out of control?

We answer that it is the person who projects his inner restraints and believes them to be imposed from without—not the person who is conscious that restraint is internal—who engages in socially harmful actions, who cheats when he thinks no one is looking, who becomes bestial in the anonymity of a mob. In the extreme case, he may project all of his inner restraints and rebel against the aggregate. Such individuals—psychopaths—do indeed require the short chain or its functional equivalent.

In contrast, a man capable of perceiving the scope of his freedom of choice necessarily perceives many other things about himself. He is in all probability a person who is aware of his ambivalent desires and capable of direct need satisfaction. He therefore has little incentive for the senseless destruction engendered by jealousy, greed, righteous wrath, and all of the other misguided motives which are spawned by misdirection and self-deceit.

In the absence of misdirection, man has no reason to act on his antisocial potential. Once a child has been socialized, the basic restraints on his behavior lie within. The self-image the adult seeks to maintain is a social product, reflecting social values, and it is to preserve this self-image that a man refrains from certain actions. This is a powerful motivation, for violation of major elements in the self-image renders self-acceptance almost impossible, and is a form of self-destruction.

The man who has an enlightened awareness of his self-interest thus sets the limits to his behavior that are necessary for self-acceptance, and it is unlikely that his choices will be very harmful to others. On the contrary, he has strong motives to seek warm relations with others, for he has a basic need for association. Aware that he chooses his actions, he does not chafe under prohibitions that he recognizes are self-impised, nor is he likely to sneak around the corner to violate them. They are essential to his self-image.

Man chooses. He chooses what he will do and what he will refrain from doing. Those restraints that are effective are self-imposed, and those barriers that are insurmountable are ones which he chooses not to surmount.

15

THE SELF AND THE SOCIAL ORDER

The member of a primitive clan might express his identity in the formula "I am we"; he cannot yet conceive of himself as an "individual," existing apart from his group. . . . When the feudal system broke down, this sense of identity was shaken and the acute question "who am I?" arose. ERICH FROMM

The normal neuroses which characterize the adjusted American are not fortuitous; most of them derive from the rise of urban-industrial society. The same transformation of society which has resulted in an unprecedented fulfillment of the physical needs has led to increased deprivation of the self needs. It is not that there are inevitable difficulties in satisfying the self needs in modern society—quite the reverse, there are unparalleled opportunities. But social change has rendered obsolete the traditional means of satisfying the self needs, and no new tradition has evolved to fulfill industrial man.

The Self in the Village
Little more than two hundred years ago, the ancestors of most Americans were European peasants who spent most of their lives coaxing food from the soil with

hand tools. In preindustrial Europe, the average man was seldom far from the line that separates subsistence from starvation, and physical needs played a greater role in his motivation than they do in the motivation of the average American. Yet preoccupation with subsistence did not mean that the peasant's self needs were deprived. He lived in a society that, for all its limitations, enabled him to satisfy his self needs in a direct and uncomplicated way.

The peasant did not find it difficult to achieve an accurate self-image. His occupation and social class established the broad outlines of his life, and these were determined by his sex and by the family into which he had been born. A boy had only to look at his older brothers and his father to predict his own future. From earliest childhood, the individual perceived clearly what he was and what he would be. Because his self-image incorporated a traditional pattern as its core, he could take what he was for granted.

It is difficult to find an analogue in contemporary society, but nationality may be one area where the American takes himself for granted in a similar fashion. He knows that there are Frenchmen and Germans and Russians, but he cannot conceive of *himself* as being anything but American. He simply *is* American. (For comparison, think of his immigrant ancestors for whom nationality was a matter of conscious choice and deliberate effort.)

The peasant had a similar sense of inevitability regarding his total self. He had only a limited awareness of other ways of being; illiterate and untraveled, he lived within horizons bounded by his fields, his village, and the nearest market town. He knew that others lived differently, but they were not potential models for him. He might envy the aristocrat (or hate him), yet he could not imagine such a life for himself. He believed that each man was born to a station in life according to the inscrutable will of God—and there the matter ended. Unable to think of himself as being anything but what he was, he had little difficulty in self-acceptance.

The same factors that facilitated ready self-acceptance also facilitated candid interaction with others. In the microcosm of the peasant village, people regarded each other as basic elements of the environment, as inevitably there as a part of the landscape. They might like or dislike each other, but dislike did not challenge the individual's right to be what he was and where he was. Personal idiosyncrasies were usualy tolerated; there was nothing else to be done about them.

For the most part, however, the peasant conformed to traditional behaviors, largely because he could not imagine behaving very differently—certainly not out of any concern about fitting into his group. He belonged in his village by birthright, as had his father and his father's father, and the rest of his ancestors. A man from a contemporary peasant village in Latin America had this kind of belonging in mind when he told us, "We are newcomers—my family has only lived here three generations." This man and his father had been born in the village and his father and grandfather had died there. But his grandfather had not been born there and by local standards these people *were* newcomers.

When a person interacts almost exclusively with people who have known him all his life, who shared his birth and breeding and will share his dying, it is impossible for him to try to maintain a false impression. The peasant assumed that friends and enemies alike knew him as he really was, and acted accordingly. He had every reason to believe that the image of himself reflected in the eyes of others was essentially valid. Being innocent of attempts to create an unrealistic public image, he could associate with others openly and candidly—and could find it easy to verify his self-image and to accept the self he experienced through association.

The peasant also possessed direct means of verifying his self-image through action. Most of his behaviors were involved with making a living, and occupation was central to his self-image. Farming was the way of life to which he was born, and few other occupations were open to him. Typically he was bound to the land by custom and by feudal law, and was not free to go into the town and learn a trade. The peasant's expectations coincided with the activities of his daily life, so he had little difficulty in expressing and verifying his self-image through his actions.

Yet the roots which nurtured the peasant also bound him. The very factors which facilitated the satisfaction of his self needs made it difficult for him to transcend the limitations of his culture. His unquestioned acceptance of a traditional self-image was matched by the fatalism with which he regarded poverty and serfdom. Such choices as he made were unencumbered by confusion about himself, but this lack of confusion was largely a reflection of his lack of self-awareness.

His consciousness of self was muted by his sense of belonging. In much the same way that a small boy learns to think of himself as "Mother's little boy" and "Mary's brother," the peasant saw himself as an integral part of a web of relationship. He was likely to answer the question "Who are you?" with a statement of lineage and kinship. He could not readily think of himself apart from his group; as Fromm has observed, the peasant tended to think "we" rather than "I." This belonging went so deep that it obscured his awareness of individual identity.

It was nearly impossible for an individual to achieve autonomy in such a society. To choose his actions and his being apart from tradition he would first of all have had to question the very foundation of his self-acceptance, to learn to imagine being other than he was, to imagine himself differing fundamentally from the kin to whom he was so closely bound. Before he could achieve the self-awareness on which autonomy is based, he would have had to break the psychological umbilical cord which tied him to tradition.

Some peasants did migrate to the cities, where since antiquity there has been a wider range of alternatives, a dilution of family ties, and a concomitant awareness of self. The city has historically drawn from the village those who were least integrated into the pattern of village life—the misfits. A rare few of these achieved autonomy in the city, but the vast majority remained simply unadjusted.

The Self in Industrial Society

Early in the period of the Industrial Revolution, social and technological change ruptured the ties of vast numbers of Europeans. The peasant who was forced off the land by enclosure acts went to the city out of economic necessity, and found that he was a peasant no longer. Suddenly he was a factory hand, counting himself lucky to have enough food to sustain life and a room to share with a dozen strangers. No less cut off from the village of their birth were those who emigrated and became American frontier farmers; such roots as these had were transplanted.

The American rural community had a homogeneity

of life style compared to the city, but it never acquired the stability of tradition which characterized the peasant villages of Europe. And, in any case, such psychic roots as the rural American had were lost when he migrated to the city. Americans have historically been a mobile people; thousands went West, and millions went to the city. At the time of the American Revolution, more than 90 percent of the population lived in rural areas. But the mechanization of agriculture released the majority of the population from food production, and the proportion of Americans on the farm is dropping steadily toward 10 percent.

Thus today the vast majority of Americans are urbanites, torn loose from nearly all of the ties that their agrarian ancestors knew. Before the Industrial Revolution, the individual drew his self-image in large measure from the traditions of the family into which he was born, and into which he brought his bride. With rare exceptions (mostly among families that have been wealthy for several generations) the American has little family tradition. The American family consists of a man, his wife, and their immature children. They have relatives, of course, but "the family" does not include them. Far from transcending the individual, this family does not even last his lifetime; every marriage creates a family and the death of one of the spouses (if there has not been a prior separation) ends it. The ephemeral modern family derives such traditions as it has from the individuals who create it; it is now the individual who gives meaning to the family, not the converse.

Nor can the typical American define himself in terms of a place. According to census figures the American family moves, on the average, once every five years. Home is where the American lives until finances permit moving up, or the job requires moving on. No one lives in the house that great-great-grandfather built. Those few who inhabit antebellum mansions or pre-Revolutionary War stone farmhouses may attempt to graft themselves onto a tradition, but the roots are not their own.

Nor can the American draw his self-image from his community. He has a sense of nationality, and sometimes an identification with a region (especially if he is a Southerner or a New Englander). This is all that remains of the identification with place of birth that formed so large a part of the peasant's self-image. Interviewing in a contemporary peasant village in Mexico, we found that the question "Where would you most like to live if you were free to choose?" was nearly meaningless. The villagers simply could not answer it. They could imagine visiting another place, but the idea of living elsewhere was puzzling. When asked where they would like to live they could only answer, "We live here." While the modern American may be sentimental about his home town, not only can he imagine living away from it, he is likely to do so by choice.

Nor does the American male have roots in a traditional vocation. The day is gone when a man could say, "We are farmers," and encompass not only himself and his living relatives but also his forefathers and his unborn descendants in a presumably eternal line. The peasant could take his occupation for granted; the role, the land he tilled, and most of the tools he used were his by inheritance. In a parallel manner, many American women have a traditional vocation. From the time that they are small girls playing house, they look forward to the day that they will be wives and mothers, and this dual role is central to their self-image. But the male child in America must decide what he will do for a living and the importance of the decision is underscored by the insistent adult inquiry "What are you going to *be* when you grow up?"

Moreover, in an industrial society in which success is considered synonymous with "making something of yourself" it is difficult for a man to find self-acceptance merely by acting out his occupational role. The idea that being successful could have any bearing on his self-definition would have puzzled the peasant. He *was* a peasant, and the size of his crop could not alter the fact. But the American finds it difficult to accept himself if he does not succeed at his chosen occupation. And in a highly competitive frame of reference, few can claim unqualified success.

Nor can the American define himself in terms of the class of his birth. Although the vast majority of Americans think of themselves as "middle class," their conception of the middle class includes many levels of affluence and prestige. The vague identification with the middle class in no way alters the American's belief that upward mobility is the measure of a man's adequacy, or his awareness of many subtle class distinctions.

In the seventeenth and eighteenth centuries, the idea that class mobility was possible was an inflammatory —even revolutionary—belief. It challenged the hereditary privileges of the aristocracy, and it opened the imagination of the peasant and the artisan to the possibility of escape from poverty. But the idea that upward mobility was possible became in time the belief that it is a requirement for acceptability; any man who does not rise above his father is considered a relative failure. This is one of the unquestioned assumptions of American normalcy, and it effectively prevents all but the most wealthy Americans from drawing their self-image from the class into which they are born.

In short, apart from his sex, his nationality, his race, and perhaps his religion or political party, there is little that the American can take for granted about himself. He is a fragment in the urban mass, not an integral part of a homogeneous community.

Yet the severing of ties that has made the American rootless has also made him self-conscious. Unable to define himself in terms of his family or his village or his social class, he is intensely aware of creating his own life and is confronted with the responsibility for what he becomes. He cannot simply drift into the expected pattern; he is forced to choose.

The individual makes a dozen minor decisions every day of his life: choosing to approach another with candor or with subterfuge, to respond with anger or with warmth, to try the new or to hang back timidly, to probe and learn or to fail to wonder when he encounters the unfamiliar. Through the choices he makes from moment to moment he shapes himself, and having done so can never fully escape the question of whether he has chosen well. In a society in which the opportunities for choice are both broad and apparent, the individual may be sharply aware that his decisions have consequences. The questions "What have I become?" and "Is it acceptable to be what I am?" have a poignancy for the American that such questions never could have had for his forebears who could simply slip into a traditional mode of being.

Thus the American—indeed, the member of any industrial society—has an intense awareness of self such as his peasant ancestors never experienced. He has, therefore, a greater need to understand and to accept himself. As industrialization has led to a gradually rising standard of living, the physical needs have become less compelling and the self needs have assumed greater relative importance in human motivation. They have also assumed a greater absolute importance, for as men have achieved heightened self-awareness their need for self-acceptance has become proportionally stronger.

The American's need to develop an accurate and acceptable self-image is intense, but his opportunities for fulfilling this need are unparalleled. He has a broad range of meaningful activity open to him and unlimited opportunity for warm and candid association with disparate individuals. He has the opportunity to exist as a conscious, articulated self to a degree seldom before realized in man's history. Adrift in an industrial society, the American is forced to choose—free to choose—and acutely aware of the self which chooses. He has an ideal situation for achieving autonomy, for being able to choose himself and his behavior in the light of his needs.

Yet it is a rare American who does achieve autonomy. Most still cling to modes of behavior which may have been functional in an earlier social order, but which are now only misdirected and neurotic patterns. Time and technology have vitiated the traditional means of achieving self-acceptance. The traditional sources of self-acceptance had the common thread of *belonging*: to family, to village, to occupation, to social class. Because the peasant belonged so unquestioningly, his awareness of choice was dulled, his sense of self was shot through with a sense of inevitability, and self-acceptance came readily. But he never *sought* to belong; belonging contributed to his self-acceptance precisely because he could take it for granted.

The adjusted American continues to associate self-acceptance with belonging. But he does not belong. Mistaking the traditional means for the end, he seeks belonging when his need is for self-acceptance. Thus he is led into conscious conformity, into trying to conceal aspects of himself which might incur the disapproval of the group where he hopes to belong. Sadly, belonging is one of those things which can never be sought successfully; one belongs only when one feels no need to seek to belong. Yet to pursue the chimera of belonging, the adjusted American sacrifices both freedom of choice and candid association, and becomes snared in the quest for indirect self-acceptance.

The peasant's birthright was group belonging, but his cultural heritage limited choice. The urban American's birthright is unlimited choice, but he spurns it for a pseudo-belonging.

Toward Autonomy

In principle, there are two routes to need satisfaction: conformity and autonomy. The individual may fulfill his needs by conforming blindly to an efficacious tradition, or he may fulfill them consciously through a deliberate choice of action.

If the society lacks an efficacious tradition, however, there is in reality only the autonomous alternative. The individual can find satisfaction only if he has sufficient understanding to make valid choices of himself, his experience, and his behavior in the light of his needs.

In a preindustrial society, blind conformity results in the fulfillment of the self needs, but also in frequent deprivation of the physical needs. Industrial society reverses this. The American can satisfy his physical needs by blind conformity, but not his self needs. The peasant can be self-accepting without being capable of autonomy; the American has an unexcelled opportunity for autonomy and an unprecedented need for it. Only through autonomy can he escape the tangle of confusion and misdirection with which his society surrounds the self needs.

famy of The imagination

16
PROSPECTUS

The voice of the intellect is a soft one, but it does not rest till it has gained a hearing. Finally, after a countless succession of rebuffs, it succeeds. This is one of the few points on which one may be optimistic about the future of mankind, but it is in itself a point of no small importance. And from it one can derive yet other hopes. SIGMUND FREUD

Political, economic, educational, religious, and other social institutions reflect the demands people make of them, even when these demands are dysfunctional. Social institutions are systems through which collective action is taken, and collective action reflects the motivations of the individual participants. If the members of a society are caught up in misdirection and customarily pursue bogus satisfactions, they will shape the institutions of their society to serve these pursuits.

Conversely, social institutions exert a formative influence on the people who participate in them. An individual learns most of his modes of thought and action from his family, his school, his occupation; he is unlikely to question or to avoid misdirections which they encourage. The relation between individual problems and social problems is one of mutual causation: inadequate social institutions shape a neurotic people,

213

and neurotic people erect and defend inadequate social institutions.

The Downward Spiral?

The American economy, for example, is shaped by the misdirected drives of the people who participate in it as producers and consumers, and in turn it trades on and stimulates these misdirected drives. Few Americans labor primarily to secure things they need or enjoy, although most are convinced that this is their motivation. Fewer still regard their jobs as a means of experiencing and enjoying their capacities. For most, the compelling motivation to work is the neurotic quest for indirect self-acceptance. In earlier chapters we have discussed the pursuit of success, recognition, and wealth as ineffective substitutes for self-acceptance. Such pursuits frequently take the form of economic activity.

There are some who see their jobs as a means of making an impressive amount of money (an incentive which is institutionalized as the "profit motive"). Some see their jobs as prestigious vehicles for rising to a higher class level, and some view their jobs as an opportunity to belong to a "team." These neurotic incentives have shaped American economic institutions. The influence of the profit motive is perhaps the most obvious, but the importance as incentives of status symbols, such as the private office, carpeted, with name on the door, and the prestige of mention in a company newspaper, or of some nominal award, has long been recognized (and utilized) by corporations. Group dynamics has become a central concept in labor relations, and the time-and-motion study is supplanted by sociograms of friendship cliques and the ubiquitous coffee break.

The output of the economy is affected by consumer

demands, and the same neurotic motives which drive the American to work influence the way he consumes. Hoping to elicit approval from others by presenting a favorably distorted view of himself, he is led to purchase products which promise to enhance his public image or to conceal his defects. The economy responds to these demands, and many goods are produced which have as their sole function embellishing or disguising the self. Even goods which have a utilitarian function (e.g., automobiles) are commonly designed and promoted as items that will enhance the buyer's prestige.

It would be an oversimplification to say that the American buys such products for gross display. There is a more subtle motive, which might be called the "Cinderella effect." Cinderella was a rejected girl until she acquired a beautiful gown and a coach and six. The adjusted American hopes that the goods he acquires will transform him in similar fashion into an exciting, desirable person. When he gets a new convertible (or she gets a new dress or a mink coat) there is an exhilarating period in which he imagines that such a transformation has taken place. The ephemeral nature of the illusion keeps him consuming.

The neurotic demands of the consumer shape the American economy, and it in turn exploits and reinforces these demands. Products running the gamut from art magazines to whiskey are hawked with the claim that they will make the person who buys them more socially or sexually acceptable to others. Some commercials apply the stick instead of dangling the carrot, and threaten that people who do not use their particular product will be social outcasts. Even soap is sold by a thinly veiled threat that people who use the wrong brand will stink.

Enticed by the promises, bullied by the threats,

and lulled by the example of compatriots who share his neuroses, the adjusted American never doubts that to be accepted and admired by others is a fundamental objective in life; nor does he doubt that he can ultimately gain this objective by consuming in such a way that he will seem to be successful, virile (or beautiful). He thinks that all he lacks is sufficient money to make such consumption fully effective. If the average American ever came to believe that he, himself—without any props—was an acceptable person, there would be some dramatic changes in the economy!

Indirect self-acceptance is pursued as insatiably by the adjusted American in his leisure as in his work. Indeed, it is during his leisure that he does much of his prestige-oriented consuming. Conspicuous consumption as Veblen described it seems to be giving way to what Riesman terms "marginal differentiation" in consumption—the art of moving ahead just far enough to excite admiration without incurring resentment. Nevertheless, much of the equipment ostensibly intended for recreation is designed and purchased as testimony to the affluence of the consumer. One need but call to mind the kidney-shaped swimming pool, the hi-fi stereo console, the automatic slide projector with synchronized tape recording—or the pink and purple sheets at Miami resort hotels—to perceive the prestige function of much that passes as recreation. To the extent that recreation has become a subcategory of the economy, directed toward the neurotic goal of impressing others, the root meaning of *re-creation* is lost.

When the adjusted American is not using his leisure to consume impressively, he is usually using it to "relax." As he understands relaxation, it means going limp in a situation which will occupy his mind just enough to keep his problems from obtruding on his consciousness. Instead of using his leisure as an opportunity for self-discovery, he seeks the means of blotting out self-awareness, of diverting his attention from a self which he has not been able to accept.

The institutional response to this quest for diversion is the entertainment industry. It offers a product which is undemanding, yet sufficiently interesting to alleviate boredom—and divert the mind from disturbing insights. It is designed to be consumed passively, to engage without requiring creative participation (and to make a profit). It trades on a neurotic flight from the self, and by insulating the individual from self-awareness, encourages neurosis.

The entertainment industry serves yet another neurotic pursuit. The adjusted American shrinks from candid association, and seeks to substitute a pseudo-intimacy based on superficial warmth and buoyed up by a froth of noncontroversial conversation. A television personality, a comic strip, or the World Series can provide material for small talk as safe as a discussion of the weather, and almost as universally applicable. The people and products of the entertainment world provide a synthetic common interest through which strangers can interact without ceasing to be strangers.

American political institutions are as influenced by normal American neuroses as are the economic institutions. Americans have many reasons for their political allegiances and attitudes, few of which have anything to do with political issues. For some, political affiliation provides a sense of belonging, particularly if their affiliation is one which is traditional in their family or region. Many people identify with a political party for about the same reasons they identify with a baseball team, and give it the same partisan support. They seek to involve themselves vicariously in an exciting contest and are ardent supporters of their "team."

For other people, political behavior is an acting out of inner conflicts. Item: a man who was denied security in childhood longs to be dependent and fears his longing. Projecting his desire to be dependent, he concludes that a lot of other people want to sit down and have someone else take care of them. Quite predictably, he is a compulsive opponent of the "welfare state" and of any politician who seems to advocate it. His opposite number is the man who finds radical political views an excellent vehicle for rebelling against his conservative family. Or there is the woman who makes a biennial penance for a secret hatred of her father by voting for the party he supported. A man joins a neo-Fascistic organization because he is attracted to the opportunities for violence and because he has projected facets of himself he would like to destroy onto Negroes, Jews, and Communists. In the ranks of any political party there are few whose allegiance is predicated on a rational decision. People offer numerous and plausible explanations for their political convictions, but these "good reasons" were discovered long after their convictions were established.

Such irrational motives for political behavior are reflected in the political institutions. Campaign managers are realists, and that part of a presidential campaign which is directed at the party regulars consists largely of tactics to reinforce group solidarity: buttons and beanies, slogans and chants, and rhythmic clapping at gatherings which have all the spirit and spectacle of a high school rally before the big game. Beyond this, little consideration is given to the party regulars who can be presumed to be committed in advance. Most of the campaign is aimed at the apathetic voter, the "independent" voter, and the possible defector from the opposition party.

The politically apathetic are for the most part people who find other outlets than politics for their inner conflicts. They may, for example, harbor racial or religious prejudices or jingoistic fervor. It is a common campaign tactic to channel such hatreds or fears into political support.

The "independent" voter claims to evaluate men apart from party labels, and regards himself as free to make the best choice. There are undoubtedly some who do so. In practice, however, the independent voter's choice usually turns on the personality of the candidate, not on his program (a fact widely recognized by campaign managers). The personality most appealing to the male voter is one which is essentially an idealized image of himself: one which combines attributes he recognizes in himself and can identify with in the candidate, minor quirks that he is fond of defending in himself, and qualities which he has alienated but longs to possess. Sometimes the candidate who can elicit such projections is a hero figure, sometimes a father figure, but in either case his essential appeal lies in those qualities which the voter projects onto him and admires tremendously.

The woman voter makes a similar identification with the candidate's wife—hence the importance of *her* public image. Having identified with the politician's wife, the woman voter judges the candidate in terms of her image of an ideal husband. The male political personality that is most appealing to her is one that she considers a romantic ideal—with a few fatherly overtones. Ardent and devoted women supporters of a male candidate resemble adolescent girls infatuated with a movie idol, for the simple reason that the same pattern of projection and adoration is involved.

The political institution is shaped by—and utilizes —these neurotic patterns. The campaign is designed to elicit such positive projections. First names and nicknames are used to give an aura of warmth and to suggest intimate acquaintance with the candidate and his wife—and thus to facilitate identification with them. Not long ago, every presidential hopeful was photographed on his farm—sometimes a recently acquired one—because the rural image was still regarded with warm nostalgia by the urban population and the farm and small-town population could identify with it. It would appear, however, that the suburban estate and the summer place are supplanting the farm as a background for the candidate, and that it is no longer necessary to minimize his wealth. (Younger voters are often puzzled to learn that Franklin D. Roosevelt's political foes delighted in portraying him as a rich man with a tall silk hat to symbolize his upper-class background.)

The inverse technique is to portray the opposing candidate in a manner that will invite negative projections. This is the smear attack which (while toeing the letter of the libel laws) manages to imply that anyone who supports the opposing candidate is either a dupe or is himself undesirable—or un-American. Such insinuations are an attempt to make the voter reject any identification with the opposing candidate, or at least be reluctant to support him openly.

The American political party exists to nominate and to elect a slate of candidates, not to formulate national policy. Thus its function is to put forward men whom the voters will accept—and it is therefore highly responsive to the voters' neurotic patterns. If the men who are ultimately elected through this process are qualified to lead the world's most powerful nation through years of crisis, it is largely by coincidence. Yet these are the men who take office, who in time do formulate policy, and who must lead the country. Because they are dependent for their tenure in office on the irrational motives of their constituents, however, they can lead only in directions which are consistent with common neurotic desires. Thus the political institution begins by encouraging the irrational and neurotic motives by which it manipulates the voter, and ends by being unable to transcend these motives.

Even the religious institutions are influenced by the neuroses common to their communicants. An increasing number of Americans are participating in the religious institutions, and in part this is a reflection of simple conformity. To a considerable degree, however, this reflects the adaptation of modern religious institutions to the neuroses and misdirections of the adjusted American. Modern religion has become nearly as bland as the entertainment industry with which it competes. And, like the major political parties, the predominant churches profess little which could make anyone uncomfortable. Gone is the longing of the finite and imperfect for the Infinite and Perfect; gone is the preoccupation with grace and salvation. Gone is the God of Wrath. In His place is the God of Love. To please his congregation, a minister may allude to Somebody Up There who accepts them in spite of their defects, and will let them belong in Heaven—provided that they observe the middle-class virtues. Perhaps the religious quest has become the search for Ultimate Indirect Self-Acceptance.

The American tradition of religious dissent has been replaced by religious conformity. (One indication of this is the number of mergers of sects which once had sharp doctrinal differences.) Theology seems to concern only the most intellectual ministers—and atheists. Perhaps in reaction to the depletion of content, there is a trend toward more elaborate forms, toward a more liturgical religion. (Familiarity with ritual has symbolized belonging since the first primitive rites were explained to young boys in puberty initiation ceremonies.) In such a setting the individual can submerge himself in ritual—and escape from self-awareness meanwhile. Thus the modern religious institutions have come to reflect the adjusted American's misdirected desire to evade self-scrutiny and his neurotic quest for indirect self-acceptance. And in turn the religious institutions encourage these normal neuroses by seeming to sanctify them.

The American family is no less influenced by neurotic patterns. It is founded on romantic love and on the search for indirect self-acceptance. The adjusted American seeks in marriage that which it cannot offer —a working substitute for self-acceptance—and often fails to find the mutual need satisfaction that marriage can facilitate. Stripped of many of its early economic and social functions by industrialization and urbanization, and called upon to fulfill an impossible emotional function, the American family founders in conflict.

The family is the least centralized and the most intimate of social institutions, and in it the next generation is shaped. Patterns of projection bind parent and child into a close but hardly salubrious relationship. Rare is the parent who is able to set an example of effective, autonomous living for his child. Almost inevitably, the child is inculcated with the neurotic patterns of his parents long before he is able to resist. Nor is it simply a matter of imitation. The actions of the average parent virtually force the child into neurosis.

For example, recall the discussion of indirect self-acceptance in chapter 6. The adjusted-middle-class-American parent makes it clear to his child from the outset that there are things he must not do and thoughts he must not think if he is to be acceptable. Unfortunately, most of these tabus reflect inevitable thoughts, feelings, and actions which the parent forbids to the child because he is terrified of such potential in himself (for example, masturbation, lying, cruelty). The parent holds up to the child an image of acceptability which derives from arbitrary propriety (and from his own attempts at self-deceit), not from any insight into human nature. The result is that, as the child discovers his ambivalent desires and potential, he is convinced that he is different from other people—and bad.

Along with the child's emerging self-image thus comes the conviction that the self he is discovering is in crucial ways inadequate or even loathsome. At this point the child falters, and the parent holds out love as a substitute for the self-acceptance which he has put beyond the child's reach. The child seizes on this substitute and struggles to keep it by concealing many facets of himself. This early inculcation of a neurotic desire for parental love and approval (as opposed to understanding) launches the child on his fruitless quest for indirect self-acceptance. And thus the family perpetuates the neuroses that shape it.

The educational institutions reinforce the neuroses the child acquires from the family. The much criticized "life adjustment" emphasis in the modern school is not a bad idea on its face. But, as developed in the usual curriculum, it becomes instruction in techniques of adjustment to conventional patterns. The child learns how to appeal to a date or how to conduct a meeting; he learns nothing of himself. The typical teacher is not trained to know himself and can hardly lead others to self-knowledge. In the aftermath of concern over such courses, however, it should be recalled that they exist in response to the demands of parents. The parent who seeks indirect self-acceptance himself wants his child well schooled in techniques of fitting in, getting ahead, and pleasing others. He demands that the school train his child in these behaviors.

In the final analysis, individual problems cannot be separated from social problems. When millions of people are caught up in misdirected efforts that lead only to exhaustion, they have neither energy nor attention to devote to the problems of their society, however great their stake in these problems may be. What attention they do pay to social issues consists largely of acting out internal problems in the social arena. And as they do, they shape the institutions of their society to serve their neurotic desires until ultimately the institutions themselves falter.

The most marked change in American institutions within recent decades is the emergence of a large and powerful military institution. This institution is new to a peacetime America, but has already become an integral part of the social structure. This is evident from the great economic stake that many communities (and even entire states) have in military contracts and installations. As Dwight D. Eisenhower stated in his Farewell Address: "This conjunction of an immense military establishment and a large arms industry is new in the American experience. The total influence—economic, political, even spiritual—is felt in every city, every statehouse, every office in the Federal government."

This new institutional complex has already begun to shape and be shaped by the neuroses of the average citizen. The faint but chronic sense of rage which characterizes the unsatisfied individual leads him to accept the thought of destruction with some relish. The idea that he might have a submerged desire to dismember and mutilate another human being may fill him with horror, but he can contemplate with jingoistic zeal the dumping of jellied gasoline on a village suspected of harboring Communist guerrillas. It has long been established that weapons are a symbol of potency for men who feel inadequate (and what phallic symbols modern missiles are, replete with warheads and measured in terms of thrust!). The average man is fascinated with these instruments and has some desire (recognized or not) to see them used.

However much he may consciously recoil from the idea, the American finds thermonuclear war increasingly credible. This is largely a result of the efforts of the public relations departments of the various military branches, who make war credible to the public in order to justify their appropriations. Dwight Eisenhower's warning has been little noted: ". . . we must guard against the acquisition of unwarranted influence whether sought or unsought, by the military-industrial complex. The potential for the disastrous rise of misplaced power exists and will persist."

Thus the world drifts toward war, carried along by the momentum of institutional development and individual neurosis, which are both tending in the same fatal direction. To justify its existence, the great military-industrial complex continues to expand and elaborate weapons systems (and not only in America). At the individual level lies neurotic motivation: the needful man feels angry, and the angry man welcomes destruction. The end will presumably come with a thermonuclear holocaust (the literal meaning of holocaust is a sacrifice wholly consumed by fire). The downward spiral in which neurotic people create social institutions to mirror and implement their misdirected desires, and in which these institutions in turn perpetuate the neuroses and use them to manipulate the people, will then have reached an irreversible bottom.

An Ascending Spiral?

A spiral can also be upward. Increased self-understand among the people of a society would be reflected in their social institutions, and living within ameliorated institutions would encourage further advances in self-understanding. If enough people became autonomous, the effect could be to accelerate the upward spiral at a geometric rate of increase. Behavior conducive to autonomy would gradually become conventional, and each successive generation could begin with more adequate patterns of living. As the retreat from autonomy tends to be self-perpetuating, so could an advance toward it.

Traditionally, it has been assumed that there is an inevitable conflict between the individual and society. Yet on analysis every instance of such conflict seems to fall into one of two classes: either the individual is confused about the nature of his self-interest, or else the society is not constituted to serve its members adequately. Increased self-understanding in the first instance and social reform in the second would be capable of removing the conflict.

Material abundance is nearly attainable today, and automation plus cheap fusion or solar power may provide the means of producing all the goods men require. There are in the world millions of half-starved people living in shacks made of cornstalks, cardboard boxes, or whatever other waste materials they can gather, but not because man lacks the technological ability to feed and house them, or the medical knowledge to treat their diseases and control their birth rate. The failure lies in faculty social organization and the individual neuroses which reflect and augment it.

A social order is conceivable in which men might resolve internal conflicts internally, instead of acting them out socially. In such a society there would be no reason for hatred among individuals or groups, for negative projections would be rare. Rather, men would be bound together by each man's need for warm and candid association. With material abundance and emotional insight, men would have little incentive to harm others, and most crime could disappear through lack of motive. Science fiction writers (the utopian writers of our time) are beginning to describe such societies, and their accounts are provocative and plausible.

In a society of the autonomous, it would be possible for social institutions to be directed toward facilitating the satisfaction of bona fide human needs. Perhaps equally important, institutions could be revised and shaped by rational decision as circumstances required. Peace within could lead to peace without, and war could be only an evil memory from a barbaric past.

At the outset, a change toward autonomy would not have to be a mass movement; autonomous individuals wield a good deal of influence on those around them. Moreover, since the autonomous can choose their actions in terms of objective reality, they frequently arrive at a consensus and act more or less in concord. Above all, they are able *to act* constructively, rather than merely to react to inner compulsions. Thus, if even a relatively small minority of Americans achieved autonomy, they might initiate an ascending spiral. And there is hope that a growing number of Americans are groping toward autonomy. In Kafka's phrase, "from a certain point onward there is no longer any turning back. That is the point that must be reached." [1]

Admittedly, all of this is a utopian dream, in which autonomy is seen as a panacea. Yet at every turning point in history there is a dream, and some panacea is seen as the way to implement it. Two hundred years ago, the utopia was a democratic society and the panacea was universal education. It seemed logical that the ills of society were a product of the ignorance of the majority. If only the masses could be educated and given a voice, it was urged, man's essential rationality would come into play, and the enlightened populace would create a truly democratic utopia. This was the vision of Locke and Jefferson. Popular education became a fact, and the masses—no longer illiterate or grossly ignorant—failed to create utopia. The ultimate disillusionment came when the most highly educated nation of the day followed Hitler into the Third German Reich. The panacea had been applied, and what ensued was hardly utopia.

A similar story could be told of other panaceas and other visions of utopia: *laissez-faire*, woman suffrage, and so on. But it is not our purpose to sketch the sad fate of past dreams. The point is that there is usually one crucial change which men hope will set in motion a chain of events leading to the solution of the basic problems of the individual and society. Later generations, having the advantage of hindsight, explain why the dream was doomed—and seek a new panacea to implement their own vision of utopia.

But even if the achievement of widespread autonomy failed to bring a utopian society, the gains would have been worth the struggle. The panaceas of the past did not lead to utopia, but most of them accomplished a great deal else. Mass education did not ensure rational behavior, but it contributed to the full development of industrial society. Autonomy is a goal worth seeking if it provides no more than a fuller life for the individual who achieves it.

And, at this turn of history, the problem is not primarily how to create utopia but, more urgently, how to prevent the destruction of civilization, perhaps of all life on earth. The American people are slowly grasping the probability of annihilation. Some are groping for a means of reversing the drift to destruction by seeking a way to disarmament. Others have burrowed into the earth in an effort they suspect is futile, shrilling that they will shoot any neighbor who tries to join them on Judgment Day. Most worry occasionally, but for the most part flee from their concern with the rationalization that nothing can be done. Still others twist their apprehension into the pretense that the only enemy is the American Communist (a label they hang on anyone who seems a safe target for the savage anger their fear has become). Some who have been passively discontent, filling empty lives with televised violence, are now moved by darker visions and turn toward potentially Fascist groups, shouting that it is treason to fear war.

If man is to refrain from genocide, it will be because the people who are able to achieve some measure of autonomy—and the rationality and objectivity which accompany it—are able to make their influence predominate. If the autonomous prevail and man learns to satisfy his needs in the industrial society he has created, he might indeed construct utopia. But if neurosis and misdirection prevail, the end is probably at hand. There seems to be a forced choice between utopia and doomsday.

NOTES

INTRODUCTORY QUOTATION

Friedrich Nietzsche, *Beyond Good and Evil*, George Allen & Unwin Ltd., London.

CHAPTER 1: THE CONFORMIST IN AMERICA

Opening quotation. C. Wright Mills, *The Power Elite*, Oxford University Press, New York, 1957, p. 318.

1. Alexis de Tocqueville, *Democracy in America*, tr. Phillips Bradley, Alfred A. Knopf, Inc., New York, 1951, Vol. I, p. 267; Vol. II, p. 332.
2. Louis Wirth, Preface to Karl Mannheim, *Ideology and Utopia*, Harcourt, Brace, New York, 1936, p. xxiv.
3. David Riesman with Nathan Glazer and Reuel Denney, *The Lonely Crowd: A Study of the Changing American Character*, Yale University Press, New Haven, 1961 (abridged edition), p. 260.

CHAPTER 2: THE SQUIRREL CAGE

Opening quotation. Lewis R. Wolberg, M.D., *The Technique of Psychotherapy*, Grune and Stratton, Inc., New York, 1954, p. 679, by permission.

1. This parable was suggested by George A. Young, Jr., M.D.

CHAPTER 3: THE MAINSPRING

Opening quotation. Ralph Linton, *The Cultural Background of Personality*, D. Appleton-Century, New York, 1945, p. 10.

1. George Bernard Shaw, *The Revolutionist's Handbook*, in *Nine Plays by Bernard Shaw*, Dodd, Mead & Co.,

New York, 1945, p. 733, by permission of the Public Trustee and the Society of Authors.

CHAPTER 4: MIRROR OF HATRED

Opening quotation. Eric Hoffer, *The True Believer*, Harper & Brothers, New York, 1951, p. 93.

CHAPTER 5: THE PERSECUTED

Opening quotation. James Baldwin, *The Fire Next Time*, Dial Press, New York, 1963, p. 18.

CHAPTER 6: INDIRECT SELF-ACCEPTANCE

Opening quotation. Eric Hoffer, *op. cit.*, p. 46.

CHAPTER 7: SOLITARY CONFINEMENT

Opening quotation. Franz Kafka, *The Great Wall of China*, trans. Willa and Edwin Muir, Shocken Books, Inc., New York, 1946, p. 264.

1. Eugene O'Neill, *Lazarus Laughed*, in *Nine Plays by Eugene O'Neill*, Modern Library (Random House), New York (n.d.), p. 457; and Richard J. Madden Play Company: Jonathan Cape Ltd., London.

CHAPTER 8: SEXUALIZATION

Opening quotation. Erich Fromm, *Man for Himself*, Rinehart, New York, 1947, p. 184.

1. George Bernard Shaw, *Man and Superman*, in *Nine Plays by Bernard Shaw*, *op. cit.*

CHAPTER 9: INTIMACY

Opening quotation. Harry Stack Sullivan, M.D., *The Interpersonal Theory of Psychiatry*, W. W. Norton, New York, 1953, p. 246, and Tavistock Publications, London.

CHAPTER 10: LOVE OR MARRIAGE

Opening quotation. George Bernard Shaw, *Man and Superman*, *op. cit.*, p. 638.

1. See Margaret Mead, *Sex and Temperament in Three*

Primitive Societies, William Morrow & Co., New York, 1935, Chapter 15.

CHAPTER 11: THE PROBLEM OF PARENTAL LOVE

Opening quotations. Friedrich Nietzsche, *Thus Spake Zarathustra*, George Allen & Unwin Ltd., London. André Gide, *The Journals of André Gide, 1889–1939*, Alfred A. Knopf, Inc., New York, 1948, Vol. II, p. 288.

CHAPTER 12: THE WEIGHT OF OBLIGATION

Opening quotations. George Bernard Shaw, *The Revolutionist's Handbook*, *op. cit.*, p. 743. Eugene O'Neill, *Mourning Becomes Electra*, *op. cit.*, p. 729.

CHAPTER 13: UNDER PRESSURE

Opening quotation. Lewis Carroll, *Through the Looking Glass*, in *Alice in Wonderland and Other Favorites*, Pocket Books, New York, 1951, pp. 144–145.

1. Erich Fromm, *op. cit.*, p. 185.

CHAPTER 14: BARRIERS AND RESTRAINTS

Opening quotation. Jean-Paul Sartre, *Being and Nothingness*, Philosophical Library Inc., New York, 1956, pp. 488–489.

CHAPTER 15: THE SELF AND THE SOCIAL ORDER

Opening quotation. Erich Fromm, *The Sane Society*, Rinehart, New York, 1955, p. 61.

CHAPTER 16: PROSPECTUS

Opening quotation. Sigmund Freud, *The Future of an Illusion*, Liveright Publishing Corp., New York. In *The Standard Edition of the Complete Psychological Works of Sigmund Freud*, tr. by James Strachey with Anna Freud, Hogarth Press, London, 1961, Vol. XXI.

1. Franz Kafka, *op. cit.*, p. 279.

INDEX